Akkon-Schriftenreihe

Akkon-Hochschule für Humanwissenschaften
Band 3

Prof. Dr. med. Dr. PH Timo Ulrichs (Editor)

Current trends in global health –

documentation and reports from conferences, symposia and workshops 2017

akkon

hochschule für
humanwissenschaften

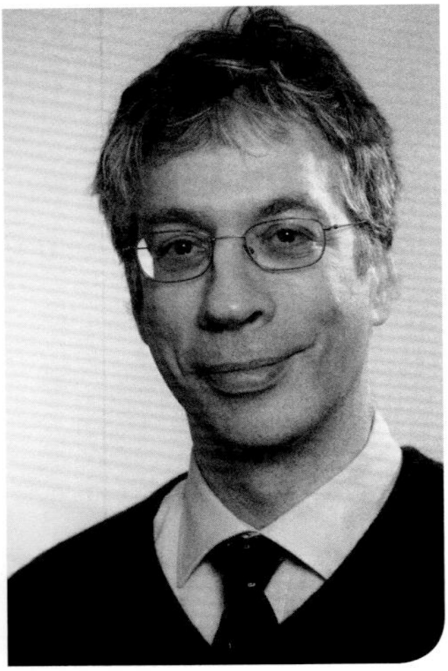

Global health is a multidisciplinary, dynamic new scientific field which primarily falls into the responsibility of the World Health Organization (WHO). However, since so many medical and health aspects also have political, economic and social impact and since many global health topics are of interest to neighbouring scientific fields such as demography, climatology, geography and political sciences, global health topics are also addressed by supranational institutions (other than WHO), national governments and facilities, non-governmental organizations, universities and scientific institutions. Their common interest is to tackle acute health issues in humanitarian aid, to elaborate suitable health strategies in development aid and to prepare the basis for future developments in human health. The current framework for all efforts in this regard is the collection of sustainable development goals (SDGs) as successors of the millennium development goals and meant to combine both environmental and development issues and to address both developed and underdeveloped countries.

The year 2017 saw a variety of conferences, meetings and workshops on various global health issues. Each topic or issue was broadly discussed by different stakeholders, and at the end of each convention, declarations, statement papers, announcements and working papers were adopted, agreed upon and published. Very often, the fate of these papers is to have a very short half-life, virtually no political or practical consequences and to be forgotten and/or replaced by new declarations or consensus papers (with the same fate).

The current third issue of the periodical of the Akkon University for Human Sciences (Schriftenreihe Band 3) is therefore published to provide current reports, summaries and documentation of global health discussions of 2017 to form a basis for future follow-up and further development. At the same time, it is also a compendium to allow the efficient use of the results of the global health discussions in 2017 for any institution to remind political decision makers of their commitments and consensus statements. The third issue has five chapters dealing with five different global health fields that played important roles in the discussions: tuberculosis, one health, humanitarian aid, the results of global health discussions at 2017's World Health Summit and global health security.

As the public and global health research network in Germany is currently being newly established under the guidance of the Robert Koch Institute (as Germany's national public health institute) and upon the initiative of the Leopoldina, Germany's national academy, the third issue of Akkon University's periodical is also meant to provide a contribution to this ongoing process and debate.

Timo Ulrichs

Prof. Dr. med. Dr. PH Timo Ulrichs,
Akkon-Hochschule für Humanwissenschaften

1. Tuberculosis as global health threat – Global and regional efforts to control tuberculosis in the year 2017

Timo Ulrichs

1.1 Introduction

Tuberculosis has accompanied mankind over millennia causing many deaths and accounting for the loss of many healthy life years from generation to generation. In industrializing countries of Europe around 1900, tuberculosis was the most prominent disease, and in the pre-antibiotic era, there was virtually no tool for a causative therapy ("therapeutic nihilism"). Then, with the development of effective anti-TB drugs in the time between the 1940s to 1960s, a combination therapy revealed to cure TB, and physicians, scientists and politicians counted on an eradication of TB within the next decade.

However, resistance against anti-TB antibiotics emerged and is now the major obstacle in efficiently control TB worldwide and especially in the WHO European Region. In fact, in 1993, WHO declared TB a global health emergency. Two developments aggravate the global TB problem in our days:

i) increasing numbers of resistances per clinical isolate of Mycobacterium tuberculosis and increasing rates of multidrug resistant cases, and

ii) HIV-TB comorbidity, especially in countries of Sub-Saharan Africa, but also as an emerging epidemic in the successor states of the former Soviet Union in the WHO European Region. In our days, the WHO European Region is the only world region with increasing rates of new HIV infections.

In order to address current challenges of TB control and to join efforts to fight the disease, a series of symposia, conferences and meetings were organized in 2017, whose major contents and results as well as impacts on research and control issues in the TB field are presented in the following chapter.

The reports cover the following symposia, conferences and meetings:

- 11th Scientific Symposium of KMF and Akkon University on the occasion of World Tuberculosis Day 2017, Berlin, March 21 and 22;
- Symposium of KMF and Central Tuberculosis Research Institute on immunological aspects of host pathogen interactions in human tuberculosis, Moscow, April 25 to 28;
- Executive Board Meeting of the Stop TB Partnership, on the occasion of the G20 Health Ministers' Conference, Berlin, May 14 and 15;

- Tuberculosis Symposium of KMF, Akkon University and Free University on the occasion of One Health Day 2017, Berlin, November 3rd, see chapter on One health, below;
- First Global Ministerial Conference "Ending Tuberculosis in the Sustainable Development Era: A Multisectoral Response" of WHO and the Russian Federation, Moscow, November 16 and 17.

1.2 11th Scientific Symposium on the occasion of World Tuberculosis Day

Berlin, March 21 and 22, 2017

"Multidrug-resistant tuberculosis in Eastern Europe – political and practical aspects of TB control"

The biggest challenge in fighting tuberculosis in the WHO-European Region is the fast growing rate of multidrug-resistant strains of M. tuberculosis in the region.

Multidrug-resistance, aggravated by an emerging HIV-epidemic in many of the successor states of the former Soviet Union, counteracts all efforts to efficiently control tuberculosis. In fact, we more and more lose control, and tuberculosis already gets virtually untreatable in some areas of our WHO-European Region. Thus, the development of new drugs and novel vaccine candidates becomes more and more urgent.

To address these challenges, Koch Mechnikov Forum (KMF) and its partners in the Russian Federation initiated scientific collaborative projects in the fields of immunology, medical microbiology, epidemiology and public health. The first scientific partnership dates back to November 2001 and is still active: The characterization of host pathogen interactions in human tuberculous lung tissue is of great importance to better understand immunological processes that are correlated with protection against infection or disease. The Central Tuberculosis Research Institute in Moscow is specialized in dissecting human lung tissue and combine human and animal model approaches. Besides immunology, various projects with partners in St. Petersburg, Smolensk, Yekaterinburg, Toms and Novosibirsk aimed and still aim at addressing problems in TB diagnostics, in case notification and infection epidemiology. KMF and its partners developed a scientific network and a variety of publications.

As a platform for scientific exchange, the symposium on World Tuberculosis Day has been launched in March 2007. The first symposium was organized to prepare the Ministerial Forum on Tuberculosis in Berlin in October 2017 which then adopted the so-called Berlin Declaration on Tuberculosis (www.euro.who.int/_

data/assets/pdf_file/0008/68183/E90833.pdf, see attachment 1). The symposia following the first year 2007 which also commemorated the 125th anniversary of Robert Koch's famous lecture "Ueber Tuberculose" each had a specific scientific focus:

2007: 125th anniversary of Koch's lecture and preparation of the Ministerial Forum and the Berlin Declaration on Tuberculosis;

2008: Current research topics in diagnostics, therapy and prevention;

2009: Public health intervention in TB control;

2010: Exchange of expertise in TB control between Eastern Europe and South Africa;

2011: Childhood tuberculosis;

2012: Evaluation of progress made in TB control four years after the adoption of the Berlin Declaration on Tuberculosis;

2013: Public private partnerships in diagnostics, therapy and prevention of TB;

2014: HIV-TB-comorbidity in different WHO world regions;

2015: Public health interventions and vaccine development; in collaboration with Tuberculosis Vaccine Initiative, TBVI;

2016: TB and migration.

Today, KMF's TB symposium on the occasion of World Tuberculosis Day is a well-established scientific meeting with both interactions among TB experts and scientists as well as with representatives of politics, public private partnerships, and other decision makers including those from WHO. The 11th symposium in March 2017 was opened by Vladimir Grinin, ambassador of the Russian Federation to Germany, highlighting the importance of joint Russian-German projects in TB control even in times of political turbulences.

State-of-the-art lectures followed, given by Lucica Ditiu, executive director of the Stop TB Partnership, about global perspectives of TB control; Martin van den Boom, WHO European Office, about the newest figures of TB in the WHO European Region; Beatrijs Stikkers, KNCV, about current aspects of TB advocacy; and Basel Karo, RKI, about the results of a study on TB therapy in the EU. The following two sessions contained best-practice examples of TB control presented by the partners of KMF in Russia, Moldova, Belarus and Moldova.

Session 4 was organized together with the Global TB Caucus (www.globaltb-caucus.org), a global organization of parliamentarians dedicated to support the fight against TB. The session was opened by the former German Federal President Christian Wulff. Members of Parliament from the United Kingdom, Saudi-Arabia and India presented their approaches to fight TB. At the end of the session, a joint declaration of the parliamentarians was presented to be submitted to the German minister of health

Hermann Gröhe, asking for integrating MDR-TB into the G20 Summit discussion of Antimicrobial Resistances, AMR. The 11th TB Symposium ended with state-of-the-art presentations on diagnostics and therapy, put forward also by private company partners such as Becton Dickinson Diagnostics and Otsuka.

Outcomes

The results of this year's 11th TB Symposium were reported directly to the World Health Summit in Berlin in October 2017 (www.worldhealthsummit.org, WHS). There, it was agreed that the political and scientific discussions will be continued in an own workshop in the upcoming WHS 2018.

The paper of the parliamentarians of the Global TB Caucus was supported by KMF and Akkon University together with many other NGOs in the field of TB research and control. It was submitted to the German Federal Minister of Health, Hermann Gröhe, who hosted the health ministers' conference of G20 in May 2017 (attachment 2).

In an open letter to the G20 member states, a consortium of many non-governmental and scientific organizations (among those the Koch-Mechnikov-Forum and the Akkon University for Human Sciences) that are active in TB research and control asked for a strong G20 statement on the necessity to strengthen efforts in fighting antimicrobial resistances and thus also TB (attachment 3).

All of these joint efforts finally resulted in highlighting MDR-TB as a major global health threat in the final document of the G20 Summit in Hamburg in July 2017 (www.g20germany.de/Content/EN/_Anlagen/G20/G20-leaders-declaration.pdf, page 9, attachment 4).

The 11th TB Symposium, the workshop at the World Health Summit and various other meetings and conferences (among those the VI. Congress of Phthisiatrists in the Russian Federation) will prepare the First Global Ministerial Conference entitled "Ending Tuberculosis in the Sustainable Development Era: A Multisectoral Response" in Moscow in November 2017.

1.3 First Global Ministerial Conference

Moscow, November 15 to 17, 2017

"Ending Tuberculosis in the Sustainable Development Era: A Multisectoral Response"

The first global ministerial conference (www.who.int/tb/endtb-sdg-ministerial-conference/en/) took place 10 years after the WHO European Ministerial Forum on TB (October 2007, which adopted the Berlin Declaration on Tuberculosis, see attachment 1) and was the attempt to widen the political support in fighting tuberculosis and thus reaching the sustainable development goals in this regard (SDG #3). The SDGs followed the millennium development goals in 2015 and combine environmental and developmental goals on the global level to be reached by 2030. Within SDG #3, the health issues are summarized, among which the fight against tuberculosis, HIV/AIDS and malaria plays an important role.

The conference was opened by the general director of WHO Tedros Ghebreyesus, by the regional director of the WHO European Region Zuzanna Jakab and the Russian Federal Minister of Health Veronika Skvortsova. President Vladimir Putin gave some welcome remarks and referred to the G20 Summit Declaration (see attachment 4), the long tradition of international collaboration in medicine and healthcare and stressed the necessity of such collaborations to reach the conference's targets.

More than 1000 physicians, scientists, political decision makers and representatives of NGOs from over 100 countries participated in the conference, among them 74 ministers. Koch-Mechnikov-Forum as a German NGO and the Akkon University of Human Sciences as a scientific institution active in the field of TB research were represented. The sessions and workshops were of highlevel quality, and the meeting with collaboration partners from other NGOs (e.g. FIND and TB Alliance), private companies (e.g. Otsuka) and partner universities and research institutes (e.g. North Western State Medical University, St. Petersburg; Central Tuberculosis Research Institute, Moscow) could be used to discuss the current joined projects and efforts in TB research.

At the end of the conference, the Moscow Declaration to End TB was adopted (www.who.int/tb/features_archive/Moscow_Declaration_to_End_TB_final_ENGLISH.pdf, attachment 5). The results of the Moscow conference also form the basis for the Highlevel UN Meeting in New York in 2018, in which the global challenges of fighting TB will be discussed on the political level.

The momentum of the political awareness of tuberculosis as a global health topic is used by Akkon University and Koch-Mechnikov-Forum by dedicating the 12th Scientific Symposium on the occasion of World Tuberculosis Day 2018 to the political framework necessary to efficiently organize global TB control efforts.

Koch-Metschnikow-Forum e. V.

Koch-Mechnikow-Forum (KMF) is a German-Russian scientific non-governmental non-commercial organisation active in healthcare realm. It was established as an initiative of the "Petersburg Dialogue" in 2006 with the purpose of contributing to aligning the Russian healthcare system with the German one. The legal framework along with the guiding priorities for its activities are enshrined in the German-Russian Agreement on Cooperation in Health signed in 2010. KMF runs projects not only in Russia, but also in a few other post-soviet states.

For over ten years, KMF has been implementing a wide range of projects and activities such as organisation of conferences, seminars, research stays, and other forms of medical and scientific exchange. Hitherto, it has successfully carried out over 150 projects on different medical topics together with its partner organisations from Russia, Georgia, Belarus, and Moldavia. Health ministries, research institutes, medical universities, health service providers, professional associations, diverse representatives of civil society, and pharmaceutical companies with social responsibility form a broad network of KMF. The work in carried out in different sections, whose heads are renown experts in their specific medicine-related fields. The main office located in the old historical building Langenbeck-Virchow House in the Berlin downtown is responsible for general coordination of projects and cross-section activities.

You can send requests to:

Prof. Dr. med. Dr. PH Dr. h.c. Timo Ulrichs
Vice-President of Koch-Mechnikow-Forum
Head of Section Tuberculosis

Address:
Koch-Metschnikow-Forum e. V.
Langenbeck-Virchow-Haus
Luisenstraße 58/59
10117 Berlin

E-Mail: timo.ulrichs@akkon-hochschule.de

Koch
Metschnikow
Forum

akkon

hochschule für
humanwissenschaften

Akkon University for Human Sciences

Akkon University for Human Sciences is a young and modern private university in Berlin, officially proved and certified. The university offers science- and problem-orientated study programs in which it reflects current sociological developments and debates. The university study program comprises education in nursing, civil protection and catastrophe relief as well as pedagogics and social sciences. Students study practically-orientated courses preparing for job positions with leadership and high responsibility afterwards. Scientific collaborations and partnerships allow professional insights into practical application of the study program contents.

Besides education and training, research and development play a major role in the overall program of Akkon University. Research projects range from basic science to applied research on practical aspects and projects commissioned to the university by governmental or private partners. In a multisectoral and interdisciplinary approach, crisis relief and resilience are central themes covered by the university.

Akkon-Hochschule für Humanwissenschaften

Colditzstraße 34–36
12099 Berlin, Germany

Tel.: +49 30 80 92 33 20
E-Mail: info@akkon-hochschule.de
www.akkon-hochschule.de

The Berlin Declaration on Tuberculosis

1. We, the Ministers of Member States in the European Region of the World Health Organization (WHO), meeting with the WHO Regional Director for Europe and high-level partners at the WHO European Ministerial Forum on Tuberculosis, held in Berlin on 22 October 2007, note with concern that tuberculosis (TB) has re-emerged as an increasing threat to health security in the WHO European Region.

- In 2005, there were 445,000 new cases of TB and 66 000 TB-related deaths in the Region.
- There are high TB incidence rates within the Region.
- Even in countries with a relatively low burden, there has been a reversal of the previous decline.
- Throughout the Region, the presence of TB is often related to social and economic factors and migration.
- Poor adherence to accepted TB control practices has created high levels of man-made multidrug-resistant TB (MDR-TB) and extensively drug-resistant TB (XDR-TB).
- No new diagnostics, drugs or vaccines have been developed over the past several decades.
- Many countries in the Region face a shortage of competent and motivated human resources for TB control.
- In the Region, TB is the most prevalent cause of illness and mortality in people living with HIV/AIDS, and few countries address TB/HIV coinfection in a comprehensive manner.
- TB does not respect borders.

2. We note that, despite some achievements over the past decade, TB control and efforts towards elimination of the disease in the Region need to be improved.

- The Region has a high proportion of unfavourable treatment outcomes resulting from poor implementation of internationally accepted TB control strategies.
- The use of currently available quality-controlled diagnostics and appropriate evidence-based treatment strategies needs to be further strengthened.
- TB control in groups at high risk such as migrant populations, the homeless, prisoners and other socially vulnerable groups must be addressed.

- Focused action is needed to tackle MDR/XDR-TB and TB/HIV coinfection.
- Prevention, including infection control, is a factor of continued importance in TB control, especially among vulnerable groups.
- Timely collection, transmission, validation and analysis of quality TB surveillance data are essential for proper TB control and elimination interventions.

1. We recognize that:

- many countries have national plans for TB control;
- a plan has been adopted to stop TB in the high-priority countries of the WHO European Region over the period 2007–2015 and a European Union action plan on TB is currently being developed;
- Member States in the WHO European Region can contribute considerably in skills and finance to the development of new tools for TB diagnosis, treatment and vaccination;
- national and international funding and support for TB activities in the European Region have grown;
- the previous United Nations Secretary-General appointed Dr Jorge Sampaio, former President of Portugal, as his Special Envoy to Stop TB;
- the Stop TB Partnership for Europe and central Asia has been launched with substantial support from the Stop TB Partnership.

2. We note with concern the gaps to be bridged in order to fully implement the Stop TB Strategy for effective TB control and agree on the following priorities:

- universal access to the Stop TB Strategy should be promoted by strengthening the health sector and involving the full spectrum of health care providers, private and public, civilian and penitentiary, all of whom should follow the International Standards for Tuberculosis Care and promote the Patients' Charter;
- civil society and affected communities should be considered as essential partners in and integrated into TB control;
- the shortfall in funds, as identified in the Global Plan to Stop TB 2006–2015, should be met through increased, properly prioritized, sustained and targeted local, national and international funding;
- TB control should be given high priority within national development plans presented for external financing;

- better use should be made of currently available effective tools, and new diagnostics, drugs and vaccines should be developed through basic research and product development, including by public-private partnerships, private industry and national research institutes;
- TB should be integrated into HIV treatment and care programmes, as the two diseases together represent a deadly combination that is more destructive than either disease alone;
- special efforts should be made to ensure that highly vulnerable documented and undocumented migrant and other populations have access to adequate culture-sensitive services providing quality care for TB;
- greater partnership and coordination across the health, penitentiary and social services sectors should be promoted, as well as inter-country collaboration.

3. We therefore commit ourselves to responding urgently to the current situation.

(i) We will strengthen:

- political will;
- the public health and social services systems;
- commitment from the full range of care providers;
- human resource capacity that is adequate in both quality and quantity for effective TB care;
- the evidence base for TB policy and practices through enhanced TB surveillance and monitoring;
- collaboration between TB and HIV programmes;
- collaboration with the private sector;
- coordination at national and international levels;
- civil society involvement.

(ii) We will adopt the Stop TB Strategy in all its components, thereby:

- ensuring the expansion and enhancement of high-quality implementation of the directly observed treatment, short course (DOTS) approach;
- addressing MDR-TB, XDR-TB, HIV-related TB and other challenges, particularly in highrisk populations;
- integrating TB care delivery with general health services and reinforcing activities aimed at strengthening health systems;

- securing commitment from all care providers;
- empowering people with TB and their communities, and removing stigma;
- allowing and promoting research into and the development of new diagnostics, drugs and vaccines, as well as programme-based operational research.

(iii) We will endeavour to secure sustainable financing by:

- implementing the resolutions on TB prevention and control adopted by the World Health Assembly in 2005 and 2007;[1]
- in collaboration with the G8 countries, supporting the Global Plan to Stop TB 2006–2015;
- attracting funding from appropriate multilateral mechanisms at the global and European levels, such as the Global Fund to fight AIDS, Tuberculosis and Malaria, UNITAID, the Bill and Melinda Gates Foundation, and other intergovernmental and philanthropic organizations, as well as bilateral mechanisms.

(iv) We will channel such financing towards:

- ensuring the implementation of regional and national plans to stop TB, including the WHO plan to stop TB in the high-priority countries of the WHO European Region;
- addressing the funding gap between the total resources available and the resources needed to control TB, as well as accelerating the development of new diagnostics, drugs and vaccines, with the aim of achieving the 2015 target related to TB within the Millennium Development goals.

1. We commit ourselves to closely monitoring and evaluating the implementation of the actions outlined in this Declaration, and call upon the WHO Regional Office for Europe, in partnership with the European Union and other relevant regional institutions and organizations, to establish adequate fora and mechanisms, involving civil society, communities and the private sector, among others, to assess progress at regional level every second year, starting in 2009.

(1) World Health Assembly resolutions WHA58.14 on sustainable financing for tuberculosis prevention and control andWHA60.19 on tuberculosis control: progress and long-term planning.

Berlin TB Summit: Outcomes Document

We, members of parliament from across the Group of 20 (G20) countries, meeting in Berlin, Germany on 20–22 March 2017, call for G20 leaders:

1. To prioritize TB within all initiatives to combat antimicrobial resistance, to ensure TB is recognised as a priority pathogen within the AMR agenda, and to devote all necessary efforts to tackling the disease within the G20 and across the world.

2. To recognize in the G20 Heads of State Declaration: the global burden of TB as the world's leading infectious disease killer; as both a cause and consequence of poverty; as a leading threat from antimicrobial resistance through drug-resistant TB; and the need to increase support for TB research and development and for the scale up and implementation of new and improved tools.

3. To establish a G20 supported mechanism to fast-track the development of a shorter and more effective TB treatment regimen, a point of care rapid molecular test and an effective vaccine which will be available and affordable for all.

Explanatory Notes

Tuberculosis (TB) is the world's deadliest infectious disease. It is airborne, drug-resistant and found in nearly every country in the world. It predominantly affects people in their most productive years, robbing children of their parents and families of their major earners. It is both a driver, and a consequence, of poverty. If we are to achieve the ambitious vision articulated in the Sustainable Development Goals (SDGs)[1] of a world free from poverty by 2030, we must first end TB.

Headline statistics on TB and drug-resistant TB (DR-TB)[2]

1. Tuberculosis (TB) is the world's leading infectious disease killer. In 2015, 1.8 million people died from TB and 10.4 million people fell ill. 4.3 million people with TB were 'missed' by their healthcare systems; that is, they were not diagnosed or treated in officially recognised settings.

2. 46 per cent (816,000) of all deaths from TB, and 54 per cent (5.6 million) of all cases of TB in 2015, were in G20 nations. The majority of these occur in Brazil, China, India, Indonesia, the Russian Federation and South Africa, but high rates are found in many other G20 countries.

3. TB is the leading cause of death among people infected with HIV and is responsible for 1-in-3 deaths from HIV (400,000). Since 2000 over 8 million people have died from TB-HIV co-infection.

4. Drug-resistant TB (DR-TB) remains a major challenge. In 2015 there were 580,000 cases of DR-TB, more than any other form of antimicrobial resistance. Overall, 55 per cent (322,000) of MDR-TB cases were in G20 countries.

TB funding worldwide

5. The World Health Organization (WHO) estimates that only US $ 6.6 billion of the US$8.3 billion required to fully fund the response to TB was provided in 2015. The majority of this funding comes from national governments, but the lowest income countries are dependent on international donors for 90 per cent of the funding for their TB programmes. Largely due to the lack of funding, the number of global cases of TB every year is falling at only 1.5 per cent a year. At this rate, TB will continue to be a threat to global public health into the next century.[3]

6 TB research and development (R&D) is critically underfunded. "The 2016 Report on Tuberculosis Research Funding Trends, 2005–2015: No Time to Lose" by the Treatment Action Group (TAG) and the Stop TB Partnership estimated that of the US$9.84 billion needed for R&D between 2011–2015 – identified by the Stop TB Partnership's Global Plan to End TB 2011–2015 – actual funding amounted to only US$3.3 billion.[45] According to the G-Finder 2016 Report only $98 million was invested in TB vaccine research in 2015 and funding for TB diagnostics research fell by 39 per cent in the last year.[6]

Market failure

7. The incentives that currently exist for commercial R&D have failed for TB. As the disease predominantly affects poor people there is little prospective financial return from new TB medicines to encourage commercial entities to make the major investments needed to develop new drugs.

8. No new drugs have entered the standard TB treatment for close to 50 years. In that period only two drugs have been developed to fight DR-TB: bedaquiline by Johnson & Johnson and delamanid by Otsuka. These drugs have both been demonstrated to improve treatment outcomes when added to treatment for DR-TB, however, it can be challenging to integrate individual drugs into existing regimens, because extensive trials are required to understand how the new combinations of drugs work together.

9. R&D for TB vaccines and diagnostics is also hampered by market failure. The current BCG vaccine was developed in 1921 and is only moderately effective in preventing severe TB in infants and young children – and it does not adequately protect teens and adults, who

are most at risk for developing and spreading TB. The majority of diagnoses of TB today rely on technology and techniques pioneered in the 19th century.

TB and AMR

10. One-third of all deaths worldwide from AMR are due to DR-TB. Experts have estimated that, in a worst case scenario, an additional 75 million people could die as a result of DR-TB by 2050. Of these, 33 million would be in the G20. The cumulative economic impact of these deaths could equal US$16.7 trillion, of which US$10.5 trillion would be in the G20. The Gross Domestic Product (GDP) of sub-Saharan Africa could be 3.21% lower in 2050 as a consequence of DR-TB, and in low-income countries as a whole it could be 2.45% lower.[7]

11. DR-TB is driven by a combination of market failure and sub-standard TB care and prevention programmes. Due to the lack of development of new and better drugs, the current treatment for drug sensitive TB requires patients to take four different types of medicines associated with strong side effects over six months. This is a major driver of the DR-TB epidemic: patients struggle to finish the full treatment course and therefore are at risk of developing resistance. Treatments for DR-TB are even more difficult than drug sensitive TB, with a very low success rate.

12. TB efforts continue to be limited by a lack of implementation and scale-up of currently available TB tools in countries. Of the 10.4 million people with TB in 2015, only 6.1 million were reached with TB care, resulting in 4.3 million being missed.[8] Only 1-in-5 people who needed treatment for MDR-TB in 2015 received it, and only half of those starting MDR-TB treatment were cured. Many high-burden TB countries are underutilizing effective new tools in the fight against TB, including rapid diagnostic tests such as GeneXpert, and new treatments for MDR-TB such as bedaquiline and delamanid.

The role of the G20

13. Leaders at the Hangzhou G20 Summit agreed that AMR "poses a serious threat to public health, growth and global economic stability," and committed to exploring options to prevent and mitigate resistance from a "G20 value-added perspective."9 As the source of the majority of public funding for medical research and development, and home to nearly all the world's major pharmaceutical companies, G20 countries are well-positioned to address the market failure that hampers antimicrobial R&D – and through carefully tailoring the intervention, could generate a significant value-add for their existing R&D efforts.

14. G20 nations are home to over half of the global TB burden. If the G20 oversees a dramatic scale-up in investment to tackle the disease, in line with the strategies above, millions of lives could be saved with existing tools. To eliminate the disease and achieve the SDGs, however, new drugs, diagnostics and vaccines must be made available to patients by 2025. To do this, the market failure hampering TB R&D most be overcome.

15. The G20 could, and should, support a new mechanism to fast-track the development of an anti-TB regimen. TB can only be successfully treated through the use of a combination of drugs, so a regimen is required. There are a number of prospective compounds already in pre-clinical development for TB, but progress has been hampered by a lack of support for further development. With the right combination of incentives, these compounds could advance relatively quickly.

16. Any mechanism should be driven by the principles of affordability, effectiveness, efficiency and equity. Where significant public funding is invested in unlocking new R&D efforts, these products should be considered as a shared responsibility and as public goods and all efforts made to ensure access and provide appropriate stewardship. Efforts must be made to incentivise knowledge sharing, collaboration and the trialling of combination of drugs as early as possible. In this perspective, we support innovative initiatives such as UNITAID that fosters innovation, fast-tracks access and reduces costs of new and more effective medicines. Such an approach will lead to faster development of a new regimen and help to ensure that all new products are accessible, affordable and appropriate for all.

17. Such an approach would serve to coordinate existing efforts to develop new drugs for the disease, ensure any new drugs developed by these mechanisms reached patients as quickly and safely as possible, and have an immediate and tangible impact on the health of people across G20 countries and around the world.

(1) Sustainable Development Goals: http://www.un.org/sustainabledevelopment/sustainable-development-goals/ accessed 01/03/17

(2) All data taken from the World Health Organization Global TB Report 2016: http://www.who.int/tb/publications/global_report/en/ accessed 01/03/17

(3) See 2 above

(4) Treatment Action Group's "2016 Report on TB Research Funding Trends, 2005-2015: No Time to Lose: http://www.treatmentactiongroup.org/tbrd2016 accessed 01/03/17

(5) Stop TB Partnership's "Global Plan to End TB 2011-2015" http://www.stoptb.org/global/plan/plan1115.asp accessed 01/03/17

(6) G-Finder 2016, Policy Cures, http://www.policycuresresearch.org/g-finder/ accessed 01/03/17

(7) Extracted from a report prepared by KPMG LLP in the UK, derived from research commissioned by the Wellcome Trust, as part of an independent review into anti-microbial resistance supported by the Department of Health and the Wellcome Trust

(8) See 2 above

(9) G20 Leaders' Communique Hangzhou Summit: http://www.g20chn.org/English/Documents/Current/201609/t20160906_3395.html accessed 01/03/17

Open letter to the G20 –

Global Health Innovation and Sustainable Development

Dear G20 Leaders and Sherpas, We are a group of like-minded organisations inspired by the German Government's prioritisation of global health during its G20 Presidency. Formed by a core group1 focused on highlighting the role of global health innovation in, for and by the G20, our inclusive coalition continues to grow and build on the momentum created during the first half of 2017.

Following the G20-focused high-level roundtable in Berlin on 28th April 2017, "Research for Impact and the G20: How can global health innovation drive sustainable development?" experts and stakeholders in attendance called on G20 leaders to play a driving role in promoting sustainable and innovative solutions to the growing crises of antimicrobial resistance (AMR), poverty-related and neglected diseases (PRNDs) and pandemic preparedness and response. Outputs from the roundtable include a Call to Action, signed by over 100 individuals and organisations, which was sent to the G20 Ministers of Health-, Development- and Research and Heads of State, and a meeting Rapporteur's Report, which outlined the presentations and discussions which took place on that day.

As the G20 continues to position the 2030 Agenda for Sustainable Development as a key priority and the "G20 Action Plan on the 2030 Agenda for Sustainable Development" is adapted to reflect updated priorities, we welcome the "Berlin Declaration of the G20 Health Ministers: Together Today for a Healthy Tomorrow". We agree that the G20 must lead by example in areas such as global health crisis management, Health Systems Strengthening (HSS) and AMR and subscribe to the focus in the Declaration on R&D for new and improved quality medicines, vaccines and diagnostics.

We appreciate the mention of several from our core group in the Health Ministers Declaration (Unitaid, CARB-X, TB Alliance, and CEPI) and the explicit mention of product development partnerships (PDPs).

We recommend that the G20:

1. Ensure that HIV, TB, Malaria, and NTDs, are included as key pathogens in urgent need of R&D under AMR.

2. Endorse the issues underscored in the Declaration and discussed at the Berlin roundtable, including the leadership of WHO in coordination and prioritization; the need for sustainable funding; the importance of Target Product Profiles (TPPs); HSS—including regulatory strengthening and

facilitating access;—and effective international R&D coordination, monitoring, evaluation and data.

3. Increase and mobilize political and financial support for global health R&D and encourage private sector and philanthropic organizations to address the inter-related issues of AMR, pandemic preparedness/response and PRNDs, as stated in the Call to Action.

4. Together with partners, continue to urge G20 Ministers to endorse our position and build on our collective message to ensure the continued prioritisation of health in, and by, the G20, to recognise the critical role of innovation, and support the prominence of health in the upgraded G20 Compact with Africa.

5. Become a regular forum for ministerial dialogue on action required to tackle serious health threats to global security and economic development and encourage G20 Leaders to reflect the critical importance of the Berlin Health Ministers Declaration in the Hamburg Leaders' Declaration.

We believe that with effective public private partnerships in global health, more rapid progress can be made in a shorter period to achieve several of the goals in the 2030 Agenda for Sustainable Development. As the G20 affirms its role in strengthening the political support for long-established and recent initiatives and continues to view its value through multiple lenses including those of economy and security, we stand by the commitment of G20 Health Ministers to continue this dialogue on global health under the Argentinian G20 Presidency.

Background and Objective of the G20 Global Health Innovation Initiative

The core group that co-hosted the Berlin roundtable "Research for Impact and the G20: How can global health innovation drive sustainable development?" is well placed to continue to highlight the role of innovation, in all forms. We continue to welcome additional members to our diverse coalition as we move this dialogue forward. The roundtable involved high-level participation by representatives of the German Bundestag, public-private partnerships, representatives of countries, including several from the G20, the private sector, academia, NGOs, the African Union, the World Health Organisation Special Programme for Research and Training in Tropical Diseases (WHO-TDR), the European Commission, together with representatives of the German Federal Ministry for Research and Education (BMBF) and the Business20 (B20) Sherpa. The roundtable discussions are summarised in the Rapporteur's Report.

We will continue to promote an open exchange with the Official Engagement Groups of the G20 and view the work of the B20, Science20 (S20), Civil20 (C20) in health as having high value. We are particularly appreciative of the strong relationship we have established with the B20 and endorse the recommendations of the B20 Health Initiative. We additionally endorse the Think20 (T20) policy brief "SDGs and health: A vision for public policy". In our "Call to Action" we formulated four recommendations leading up to the G20 Health Ministers Summit. Over 100 public and private stakeholders supported these recommendations and strongly agreed that the G20 should become a regular forum for ministerial dialogue on action required to tackle these serious health threats to global security and economic development. As global health advocates, we are appreciative of the impact of our initiative and we see high value in building on this with your support. We wish you a successful meeting.

Signed by Organisations:

Global Health Technologies Coalition (GHTC), PATH, CEPI, Sabin Vaccine Institute, Unitaid, Medicines for Malaria Venture, Sovereign Strategy, TB Alliance, Columbia University, International Rescue Committee, Koch-Metschnikow-Forum, AMR Centre, IntraHealth, AERAS, Treatment Action Group, Akkon-Hochschule für Humanwissenschaften, International Vaccine Institute, Washington Global Health Alliance, FIND, Global Health Innovative Technology Fund (GHIT), TuBerculosis Vaccine Initiative (TBVI), King Saud University, Policy Cures Research, Wits Reproductive Health and HIV Institute (WITS RHI), American Society of Tropical Medicine & Hygiene (ASTMH), The Amsterdam Institute of Global Health and Development (aighd), International AIDS Vaccine Initiative (IAVI), Elizabeth Glaser Pediatric AIDS Foundation, The Leprosy Mission, The London Centre for Neglected Tropical Disease Research, Liverpool School of Tropical Medicine (LSTM), BioMérieux, The International Union Against Tuberculosis and Lung Disease (The Union), International Coalition for Trachoma Control (ICTC), MedTech Europe

Signed by Individuals:

Jeremy Lefroy MP, UK Member of Parliament, Chair of the Parliamentary Network on the World Bank and International Monetary Fund

MdB Kordula Schulz-Asche, Member of the German Bundestag

John Bowis, Former UK Health Minister, Hon President Health First Europe

Rajae El Aouad, MD, MSc, MHPM, Member of the Hassan II Academy of Science and technology of Morocco

Councillor Julie Donoghue, Rushcliffe Borough Council, UK and member of the All Party Parliamentary Group (APPG) for Malaria and Neglected Tropical Diseases

Professor Janet Hemingway, Director of Liverpool School of Tropical Medicine; Chair in Insect Molecular Biology

Richard Feiner, Columbia University

Dra. Rosa María Herrera Torres, MD TB survivor

Prof. Dr. med. Dr. PH Dr. h.c. Timo Ulrichs, Head of Programm, Internationale Not- und Katastrophenmedizin Akkon-Hochschule für Humanwissenschaften, Vice-President and Head of the Tuberculosis Section of the Koch-Metschnikow-Forum

G20 Leaders' Declaration

Shaping an interconnected world

Preamble:
We, the Leaders of the G20, met in Hamburg, Germany on 7-8 July 2017 to address major global economic challenges and to contribute to prosperity and well-being.

Mastering the challenges of our age and shaping an interconnected world is the common goal of the G20 as our premier forum for international economic cooperation. The G20 revealed its strength during the global economic and financial crisis some ten years ago when it played a crucial role in stabilising economies and financial markets. What was true then continues to hold: We can achieve more together than by acting alone.

Progressing our joint objective in the G20 – strong, sustainable, balanced and inclusive growth – remains our highest priority.

Globalisation and technological change have contributed significantly to driving economic growth and raising living standards across the globe. However, globalisation has created challenges and its benefits have not been shared widely enough. By bringing together developed and emerging market economies, the G20 is determined to shape globalisation to benefit all people. Most importantly, we need to better enable our people to seize its opportunities.

We are resolved to tackle common challenges to the global community, including terrorism, displacement, poverty, hunger and health threats, job creation, climate change, energy security, and inequality including gender inequality, as a basis for sustainable development and stability. We will continue to work together with others, including developing countries, to address these challenges, building on the rules- based international order.

Expanding on the results of previous presidencies, in particular the 2016 G20 Summit in Hangzhou, we decide today to take concrete actions to advance the three aims of building resilience, improving sustainability and assuming responsibility.

(...)

20. **Safeguarding against Health Crises and Strengthening Health Systems:** The G20 has a crucial role in advancing preparedness and responsiveness against global health challenges. With reference to the results of the G20 health emergency simulation exercise, we emphasise the value of our ongoing, trust-building, cross-sectoral

cooperation. We recall universal health coverage is a goal adopted in the 2030 Agenda and recognize that strong health systems are important to effectively address health crises. We call on the UN to keep global health high on the political agenda and we strive for cooperative action to strengthen health systems worldwide, including through developing the health workforce. We recognise that implementation of and compliance with the International Health Regulations (IHR 2005) is critical for efficient prevention, preparedness and response efforts. We strive to fully eradicate polio. We also acknowledge that mass movement of people can pose significant health challenges and encourage countries and International Organisations to strengthen cooperation on the topic. We support the WHO´s central coordinating role, especially for capacity building and response to health emergencies, and we encourage full implementation of its emergency reform. We advocate for sufficient and sustainable funding to strengthen global health capacities, including for rapid financing mechanisms and the WHO's Health Emergencies Programme. Furthermore, we see a need to foster R&D preparedness through globally coordinated models as guided by the WHO R&D Blueprint, such as the Coalition for Epidemic Preparedness Innovations (CEPI).

21. **Combatting Antimicrobial Resistance (AMR):** AMR represents a growing threat to public health and economic growth. To tackle the spread of AMR in humans, animals and the environment, we aim to have implementation of our National Action Plans, based on a One-Health approach, well under way by the end of 2018. We will promote the prudent use of antibiotics1 in all sectors and strive to restrict their use in veterinary medicine to therapeutic uses alone. Responsible and prudent use of antibiotics in food producing animals does not include the use for growth promotion in the absence of risk analysis. We underline that treatments should be available through prescription or the veterinary equivalent only. We will strengthen public awareness, infection prevention and control and improve the understanding of the issue of antimicrobials in the environment. We will promote access to affordable and quality antimicrobials, vaccines and diagnostics, including through efforts to preserve existing therapeutic options. We highlight the importance of fostering R&D, in particular for priority pathogens as identified by the WHO and tuberculosis. We call for a new international R&D Collaboration Hub to maximise the impact of existing and new anti-microbial basic and clinical research initiatives as

well as product development. We invite all interested countries and partners to join this new initiative. Concurrently, in collaboration with relevant experts including from the OECD and the WHO, we will further examine practical market incentive options.

Improving Sustainable Livelihoods

22. **Energy and Climate:** A strong economy and a healthy planet are mutually reinforcing. We recognise the opportunities for innovation, sustainable growth, competitiveness, and job creation of increased investment into sustainable energy sources and clean energy technologies and infrastructure. We remain collectively committed to mitigate greenhouse gas emissions through, among others, increased innovation on sustainable and clean energies and energy efficiency, and work towards low greenhouse-gas emission energy systems. In facilitating well-balanced and economically viable long-term strategies in order to transform and enhance our economies and energy systems consistent with the 2030 Agenda for Sustainable Development, G20 members will collaborate closely. Recalling the G20 Principles on Energy Collaboration, we regard energy security as one of the guiding principles for the transformation of our energy systems, and we will continue to work on open, flexible, and transparent markets for energy commodities and technologies. We welcome international cooperation on the development, deployment, and commercialisation of sustainable and clean energy technologies and support financing by Multilateral Development Banks to promote universal access to affordable, reliable, sustainable and clean energy.

24. We take note of the decision of the United States of America to withdraw from the Paris Agreement. The United States of America announced it will immediately cease the implementation of its current nationally-determined contribution and affirms its strong commitment to an approach that lowers emissions while supporting economic growth and improving energy security needs. The United States of America states it will endeavour to work closely with other countries to help them access and use fossil fuels more cleanly and efficiently and help deploy renewable and other clean energy sources, given the importance of energy access and security in their nationally- determined contributions.

25. The Leaders of the other G20 members state that the Paris Agreement is irreversible. We

reiterate the importance of fulfilling the UNFCCC commitment by developed countries in providing means of implementation including financial resources to assist developing countries with respect to both mitigation and adaptation actions in line with Paris outcomes and note the OECD's report "Investing in Climate, Investing in Growth". We reaffirm our strong commitment to the Paris Agreement, moving swiftly towards its full implementation in accordance with the principle of common but differentiated responsibilities and respective capabilities, in the light of different national circumstances and, to this end, we agree to the G20 Hamburg Climate and Energy Action Plan for Growth as set out in the Annex.

26. **Leading the Way towards Sustainable Development:** The adoption of the 2030 Agenda represented a milestone towards global sustainable development. We call on countries to work with stakeholders to strive towards its ambitious and integrated implementation and timely realisation in accordance with national circumstances. We commit to further align our actions with the 2030 Agenda for Sustainable Development and its integral part, the Addis Ababa Action Agenda on Financing for Development, domestically and internationally, including in support of developing countries and the provision of public goods.

27. Building on the G20's Action Plan on the 2030 Agenda for Sustainable Development, the Hamburg Update emphasises our collective and concrete commitments. We support the central role of the high-level political forum on sustainable development and other key UN processes towards achieving the Sustainable Development Goals. We will also engage in voluntary peer learning on the implementation of the 2030 Agenda and call upon others to join this important exercise as a complementary action towards Voluntary National Reviews.

(...)

MOSCOW DECLARATION TO END TB

First who global ministerial conference ending TB in the sustainable development era: a multisectoral response

16–17 november 2017, Moscow, Russian Federation

Preamble

We, the Ministers of Health and from across Governments acknowledge that despite concerted efforts, tuberculosis (TB), including its drug-resistant forms, causes more deaths than any other infectious disease worldwide and is a serious threat to global health security.

TB kills more than five thousand children, women and men each day and leaves no country untouched.a It is one of the leading killers among people of working age which creates and reinforces a cycle of ill-health and poverty, with potential catastrophic social and economic consequences for families, communities, and countries. While recognizing the higher prevalence of TB among men, women and children are also vulnerable to the consequences of TB due to gender- and age-related social and health inequalities, such as poor health literacy, limited access to health services, stigma and discrimination, and exposure to the infection as carers. Multidrug-resistant TB (MDR-TB) accounts for one-third of all antimicrobial resistance (AMR)-related deaths, making the global AMR agenda central to tackling TB. TB is also the principal cause of death among people living with HIV/AIDS. The global TB targets will not be met without new and more effective tools and innovative approaches for prevention, diagnosis, treatment and care. Persistent funding gaps impede progress towards ending TB.

Although a concern to all people, TB disproportionately afflicts the poorest and the most vulnerable populations. Tobacco smoking, harmful use of alcohol and other substance abuse, air pollution, exposure to silica dust, living with HIV/AIDS, diabetes and malnutrition increase the risk of TB. Stigma and discrimination remain critical barriers to TB care.

We reaffirm our commitment to end the TB epidemic by 2030 as envisaged in the Agenda 2030 for Sustainable Development and its Sustainable Development Goals (SDGs), the World Health Organization (WHO) End TB Strategy, and the Stop TB Partnership Global Plan to End TB 2016-2020. We acknowledge that to fundamentally transform the fight against TB, we need to:

(i) address all the determinantsb of the TB epidemic including through a high-level commitment to, and implementation of, a multisectoral approach;[c]

(ii) achieve rapid progress towards the goal of universal health coverage through health systems strengthening, while also ensuring universal access to quality people-centred TB prevention and care, ensuring that no one is left behind;

(iii) implement measures aimed at minimizing the risk of the development and spread of drug resistance taking into account global efforts to combat AMR;

(iv) secure sufficient and sustainable financing, especially from domestic sources, and mobilize, as needed, additional financing from development banks, development partners and donor agencies;

(v) advance research and development, as well as rapid uptake, of new and more effective tools for diagnosis, treatment, drug regimens, and prevention including vaccination, and ensure that we translate existing and emerging knowledge into concrete action to achieve rapid results;

(vi) actively engage people and communities affected by, and at risk of, TB.

Furthermore, an effective TB response requires a global, regional, cross-border and country specific approach with multisectoral and multi-stakeholder actions, with recognition of: (i) significant differences among and within countries with high, intermediate and low incidence of TB and MDR-TB, (ii) demographic and social trends such as population ageing and urbanization, and (iii) needs of the affected individuals and communities, and the challenges in reaching and identifying all people with TB and providing them with appropriate care.

We recognize this First WHO Global Ministerial Conference, Ending TB in the Sustainable Development Era: A Multisectoral Response, convened by the WHO and the Government of the Russian Federation, as a fundamental milestone towards the United Nations General Assembly (UNGA) High-Level Meeting on TB in 2018. To fulfil the commitments and calls to action in this Declaration, and to achieve the most from the UNGA High-Level Meeting, we need to enlist the full engagement of, and collaboration among, heads of state, UN leadership and other global leaders; technical agencies and academia; private sector and philanthropic foundations; civil society and other relevant partners (such as patients groups, health professionals, social and community workers organizations and funding agencies).

Commitments and calls to action

We commit ourselves to ending TB, which is a political priority defined in the Agenda 2030 and as a contribution to achieving universal health coverage, within national legislative and policy frameworks, and to implementing the following actions through approaches protecting and promoting equity, ethics, gender equality, and human rights in addressing TB, and based on sound, evidence-based, public health principles. We urge WHO, and call upon other UN organizations and all partners, to provide the support necessary for success:

1. Advancing the TB response within the SDG agenda

We commit to

- Scaling up TB prevention, diagnosis, treatment and care and working towards the goal of universal health coverage through public and private health care providers to achieve detection of at least 90 per cent of cases and successful treatment of at least 90 per cent of those detectedd in all countries through the use of rapid diagnostics (including molecular diagnostics), appropriate treatment, patient-centred care and support, applying WHO-recommended standards of caree, and harnessing digital healthf.
- Prioritizing, as appropriate, notably through the involvement of communities and civil society and in a non-discriminatory manner, high-risk groups and populations in vulnerable situations such as women and children, indigenous people, health care workers, the elderly, migrants, refugees, internally displaced people, prisoners, people living with HIV/AIDS, people who use drugs, miners, urban and rural poor and under-served populations, without which TB elimination will not be possible.
- Addressing MDR-TB as a global public health crisis including through a national emergency response in at least all high MDR-TB burden countries, while ensuring that robust systems are sustained in all countries to prevent emergence and spread of drug resistance. Rapidly scaling up access to patient-centred, integrated TB and HIV services and collaborative activities to end preventable deaths due to TB among people living with HIV/AIDS.g [h]
- Achieving synergies in managing TB, co-infections and relevant noncommunicable diseases, undernutrition, mental health and harmful use of alcohol and other substance abuse, including drug injection.

- Working to increase, when relevant, access to new and effective tuberculosis drugs under strict programmatic monitoring and follow-up.

- Ensuring, as appropriate, adequate human resources for TB prevention, treatment and care.

- Reducing stigma, discrimination and community isolation, and promoting patient-centred care including community-based treatment options, as well as psychosocial and socioeconomic support.

We call upon

- WHO, other UN agencies, the Global Fund to Fight AIDS, TB and Malaria, the Stop TB Partnership, UNITAID, donors and partners, including from the private sector, academia and philanthropic foundations, and civil society to support the implementation of this Declaration.

- WHO, bilateral and multilateral funding agencies and other partners to urgently support high MDR-TB burden countries in their national emergency response.

- WHO, other UN agencies, bilateral and multilateral funding agencies and technical partners to address MDR-TB as a major threat to public health securityi by supporting implementation of the Global Action Plan on AMR in all countries, while we reaffirm the political declaration of the high-level meeting of the UN General Assembly on antimicrobial resistance.

2. Ensuring sufficient and sustainable financing

We commit to

- Working with heads of state and across ministries and sectors, as appropriate, to mobilize the domestic financing needed for health systems strengthening with the ultimate goal of reaching universal health coverage, in keeping with national legislative frameworks, and with the Addis Ababa Action Agenda of the Third International Conference on Financing for Development.[k]

- Developing and implementing, as appropriate, more ambitious, fully-funded national TB policies and strategic plans, including for TB research, that are aligned with national health plans, frameworks and the End TB Strategy and in keeping with national legislative frameworks.

- Identifying and implementing, as appropriate, the actions required to address issues that cause catastrophic costsl to patients and their households, to ensure social protection measures, while ensuring that actions are in line with human rights obligations.

We call upon

- Global health financing partners including the Global Fund to Fight AIDS, TB and Malaria, the Global Financing Facility, bilateral agencies, the World Bank, and regional development banks to pursue and advocate for additional financing including through blendedm and/or other forms of innovative financing, with adequate safeguards for ensuring public health impact and attention to key populations.
- WHO to continue providing strategic and technical leadership, advice and support to Member States as well as to international institutions.
- Academic, technical, civil society, private sector and other relevant partners to continue their efforts to help countries develop and pursue investment casesn while supporting health systems strengthening and increased absorption capacity.°

3. Pursuing science, research and innovation

We commit to

- Increasing national and/or regional capacity and funding, as needed, to urgently expand multidisciplinary TB research and innovation, as well as applied health research, by establishing and/or strengthening national TB research networks including civil society and community-based mechanisms, considering TB research as a central element of national TB and R&D strategies, expanding existing networks to integrate TB research, and reducing research- and implementation-related regulatory impediments.
- Working, when relevant, across ministries, donors, the scientific community and the private sector, academia, and other key stakeholders for the purpose of research: (a) for development and evaluation of (i) rapid point of care diagnostics, (ii) new and more effective drugs, and shorter, high-quality and cost-effective treatment regimens for all forms of TB (including latent TB infection and drug-resistant TB), and (iii) safe and effective TB vaccines by 2025; and (b) on environmental and social determinants of TB and effective interventions strategies.
- Improving, as appropriate, the coordination of research efforts nationally and globally, and ensuring that the emerging knowledge is promptly put into action, including by putting in place appropriate policy frameworks and implementing new medical technologies. Strengthening, as appropriate, surveillance systems, improving data collection and reporting at all levels, utilising innovative approaches and including surveillance in TB research agendas.

We call upon

- WHO in collaboration with global partners, research organizations, donors, the scientific community and countries to consider developing a Global Strategy for TB Research taking into consideration ongoing and new efforts, such as the TB Research Network stated in the BRICS Leaders Xiamen Declaration.

- WHO in collaboration with global health and research partners and countries to make further progress in enhancing cooperation and coordination of TB research and development, considering where possible drawing on existing research networks to integrate TB research, such as the new AMR Research and Development Collaboration Hub proposed in the 2017 G20 Leaders' Declaration, notably to facilitate rapid scale up of innovative approaches and tools for TB prevention, diagnosis, treatment and care.

4. Developing a multisectoral accountability framework

To end TB by 2030, we will need reliable data to ensure that our collective knowledge is transformed into effective and timely action, both globally and domestically, and that we deliver on the commitments made in this Declaration. A new multisectoral accountability framework should enable the review and monitoring of implementation and provide a systematic approach to determine additional actions required to achieve the SDG and End TB Strategy milestones and targets. The accountability framework should build upon evidence, independent analysis and constructive collaboration among all relevant partners, with an emphasis on high-burden countries, and should avoid duplication and increased reporting burden. To maximize impact, a multisectoral accountability framework that is based on approaches protecting and promoting equity, gender equality, human rights and ethics could, according to needs, include:

a) The convening of national inter-ministerial commissions on TB, or their equivalent, by Ministries of Health in partnership with civil society and, where appropriate, with the direct engagement of the Heads of State, and the consideration of expanding existing intersectoral fora to include actions against TB in consultation with existing entities the goals of which include combatting TB so as to avoid duplication of efforts;

b) Mechanisms for strengthening advocacy at all levels within all relevant sectors;

c) Well-defined reporting, including sex- and age-disaggregated data, and review processes to monitor progress toward clear goals; and

d) Opportunities for active engagement, monitoring, reporting and/or audits by civil society, as well as other key stakeholders.

We commit to

- Supporting the development of a multisectoral accountability framework in advance of the 2018 UNGA High-Level Meeting on TB, to track progress towards the SDG target of ending TB using relevant SDG indicators and the End TB Strategy operational indicators, and applying financing benchmarks set by the Stop TB Partnership Global Plan to Stop TB 2016-2020.

We call upon

- WHO, working in close cooperation with the UN Special Envoy on TB, Member States, including, where applicable, regional economic integration organizations, civil society representatives, UN Organizations, the World Bank and other multilateral development banks, UNITAID, the Stop TB Partnership, the Global Fund to Fight AIDS, TB and Malaria, research institutes and other partners, to develop the multisectoral accountability framework for the consideration of the WHO Governing Bodies, while taking into account existing multisectoral and multi-stakeholder frameworks, that enables measuring progress both globally and nationally through an independent, constructive and positive approach, especially in the highest burden countries, and an independent review of progress by those countries.
- WHO, in collaboration with Member States and key stakeholders, to develop a reporting framework and periodicity for a multisectoral global progress report on TB, subject to independent review.

Way forward

- We conclude with a commitment to act immediately on this Declaration in coordination with the WHO, and to engage with leaders and all relevant sectors of Government, UN agencies, bilateral and multilateral funding agencies and donors, academia, research organizations, scientific community, civil society and the private sector to prepare for and follow-up on the UNGA High-Level Meeting on Tuberculosis in 2018 in New York.

Explanatory Notes

a) Please see the 2016 WHO Global TB Report: http://apps.who.int/medicinedocs/en/d/Js23098en/.

b) TB determinants and/or risk factors: Conditions that favour transmission of TB or make people vulnerable to get TB are called TB determinants. The important social determinants of TB include poverty, and poor living and working conditions. Communicable and noncommunicable disease and other conditions that increase individual risk of getting TB are called risk factors. These include HIV/AIDS and other conditions that weaken the immune system, diabetes, silicosis, tobacco smoking, undernutrition, harmful use of alcohol and other substance abuse.

c) Multisectoral approach: Preventing TB or minimizing the risk of TB certainly requires not only actions by the health sector (such as achieving universal health coverage and control of communicable and noncommunicable diseases that are major risk factors for TB) but also by other development sectors (such as poverty reduction, improved food security, better living and working conditions).

d) As recommended in the WHO guidance on implementing the End TB Strategy: ttp://www.who.int/tb/publications/2015/end_tb_essential.pdf?ua=1.

e) Standards of care: WHO-recommended standards for optimum delivery of TB care and prevention, presented in the Compendium of WHO guidelines and associated standards: ensuring optimum delivery of the cascade of care for patients with TB.

f) Please see the document, WHO Digital health for the End TB Strategy - an agenda for action http://www.who.int/tb/publications/digitalhealth-TB-agenda/en/.

g) Eliminating preventable deaths among people living with HIV: This is in line with the target of reducing TB-related deaths among people living with HIV by 75 per cent by 2020, adopted by the UN General Assembly in the Political Declaration on HIV and AIDS: On the Fast Track to Accelerating the Fight against HIV and to Ending the AIDS Epidemic by 2030.

h) Please see the document, WHO policy on collaborative TB/HIV activities http://www.who.int/tb/publications/2012/tb_hiv_policy_9789241503006/en/.

i) As stated in WHA Resolution 62.15 from 2009: "Concerned that the highest levels of multidrug-resistance reported in WHO's fourth global report on anti-tuberculosis drug resistance – an estimated half a million multidrug-resistant cases occurring globally, including 50 000 cases of extensively drug-resistant tuberculosis – pose a threat to global public health security" http://apps.who.int/gb/ebwha/pdf_files/WHA62-REC1/WHA62_REC1-en-P2.pdf.

j) Please see the documents WHO Global Action Plan on AMR http://www.who.int/antimicrobial-resistance/global-action-plan/en/ (adopted by the 68th WHA http://apps.who.int/gb/ebwha/pdf_files/WHA68/A68_R7-en.pdf?ua=1), and the Political declaration of the high-level meeting of the UN General Assembly on AMR http:// www.un.org/pga/71/wp-content/uploads/sites/40/2016/09/DGACM_GAEAD_ESCAB-AMR-Draft-Political- Declaration-1616108E.pdf.

k) Please see the document, Addis Ababa Action Agenda of the Third International Conference on Financing for Development http://www.un.org/esa/ffd/wp-content/uploads/2015/08/AAAA_Outcome.pdf.

l) Catastrophic costs: The costs due to TB measure the total economic burden on TB patients and their families and are considered catastrophic when they threaten the livelihood of patients and their families. These costs include: payments for care (e.g. diagnostic and treatment services, and medicines), payments associated with care seeking (e.g. travel costs) and the "opportunity costs" associated with care seeking (e.g. lost income). These are determined by undertaking surveys of TB patients in health facilities.

m) Blended financing: Complementary use of grants (such as from the Global Fund or other donors) and non-grant financing from private and/or public sources (such as a World Bank loan) on terms that would make a programme financially sustainable.

n) Investment case: The Investment Case is a description of the transformation that a country wants to see to meet the targets and milestones towards ending the TB epidemic, and a prioritized set of investments required to achieve the results.

o) Absorption capacity: Capacity of a country health system to put a significantly increased flow of resources to efficient use, which depends generally on governance, institutional capacity, ownership, and social and political stability.

Conference website
http://www.who.int/tb/endtb-sdg-ministerial-conference/en/

Foundation of the Research Institute in International Assistance at Akkon University

Crisis, catastrophe and conflict situations increase globally, both in frequency and intensity. Crises become more and more complex, be it acute situations like earthquakes or outbreaks/epidemics or chronic catastrophes like tuberculosis or drought. To ensure the development of short-term and long-term answers and solutions to the increasing and imminent questions of humanitarian and development aid, Akkon University will found a research institute dedicated to further interdisciplinary and collaborative research in this neglected field.

akkon hochschule für humanwissenschaften

iria institute for research in international assistance

Contact

Prof. Dr. med. Dr. PH Dr. h.c. Timo Ulrichs
Akkon University for Human Sciences
Colditzstraße 34–36,
12099 Berlin, Germany
timo.ulrichs@iria.akkon-hochschule.de
www.iria.akkon-hochschule.de

The "Institute for Research in International Assistance" (IRIA) at Akkon University will focus on general questions in humanitarian and development aid and thus provide scientific basis for respective political and social debates. In particular, the institute will focus on the following urgent research questions in health:

- Restructuring global health to reach the sustainable development goal 3
- Civil-military collaboration in humanitarian and development aid
- Global health security
- Health care systems in transition, especially in Eastern Europe and Central Asia
- One Health approaches in fighting zoonoses
- Fighting (re-)emerging infectious diseases

The first projects were already started and are currently financed by third-party funding. However, IRIA will have to be co-financed by additional partners, and thus we invite you to join and support the basic idea of improving research in humanitarian and development aid!

DFG Deutsche Forschungsgemeinschaft

"The Institute for Research in International Assistance will be officially founded on the occasion of a scientific symposium in global health which will take place at Akkon University May 14, 2018, and will be funded by the German Research Foundation, DFG."

2. International One Health Day 2017 Transdisciplinary Workshop

Paulin Dettmann, Clara Schubert, Fabienne Eichler

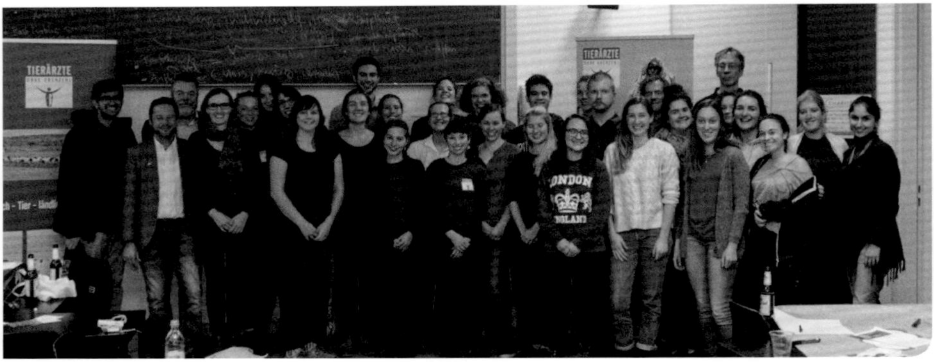

▲ *One Health Workshop Participants and speaker of the workshop 2017 (c) Reers*

Would you be surprised if someone told you that the environment has a great impact on your health? And have you ever wondered if you can transmit your cold to your beloved pet?

As volunteers for the Non-Governmental Organisation Vétérinaires Sans Frontières e. V. Germany we care about these kinds of questions. The correlation between environment and our status of health sounds logical and significant to us. In combination with learning about diseases, which can be spread between humans and animals, so-called zoonosis, we are finding ourselves in the middle of the One Health approach.

One Health's catchphrase by the American Veterinary Medical Association goes as the following: "One Health is the collaborative effort of multiple disciplines – working locally, nationally and globally – to attain optimal health for people, animals and the environment." (1)

We, the volunteers, are fascinated by the One Health approach and have made it our goal to spread its message. Consequently, we organised once more a transdisciplinary workshop on behalf of the international One Health Day 2017. It was funded by Engagement Global and the Federal Ministry for Economic Cooperation and Development (3), and for this project's implementation, students of medicine and veterinary medicine worked together. As last year's event was taking place at the Free University Berlin, the university for future veterinarians, the latest workshop was held at the Charité-Universitätsmedizin Berlin, the medical students' university. We are drawing closer together.

We have not yet answered the question if you can infect your pet with your cold. Luckily, it is unlikely. However, there are many zoonosis, which urgently need a collaborative concept of defence. The workshop's focus lied on tuberculosis as a transmissible disease, for which experts with different scientific and clinical backgrounds were invited as speakers. And, most encouragingly, the varied audience included students and professionals of medical, veterinary, public health, geography, biology and further related fields of studies.

Should veterinarians be more aware of this disease or the physicists? Since 1997, Germany has gained the bovine tuberculosis free status, but 46 new cases were reported in 2013. In comparison: there were 6000 reported cases of human tuberculosis in 2016 in Germany.

First, Ralf Otto-Knapp, an expert of the Central Committee for the Fight against tuberculosis in Germany talked about the history of tuberculosis and the development of testing methods.

Do you know the symptoms of tuberculosis in humans? Before we are answering this question, we need to differentiate between two kind of tuberculosis infections.

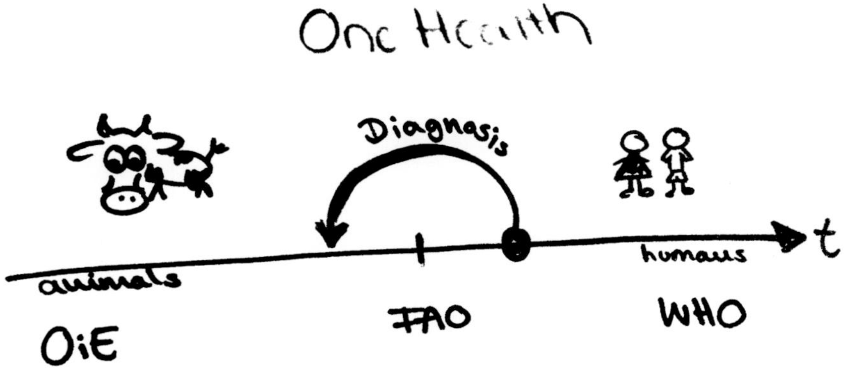

▲ *Sketch by one participant*
The One Health approach includes earlier diagnostics and collaboration of Global Health Actors, which aims to prevent the spread of diseases

Tuberculosis' causing agent in humans is Mycobacterium tuberculosis, but the type Mycobacterium bovis can be spread between humans and animals, especially cattle. It is unknown, if cattle can be infected by M. tuberculosis, too. Both, bovine and human tuberculosis are mainly spread via air droplets and mainly affect the respiratory system.

Firstly, the latent tuberculosis, of which an estimated 2 billion people are affected without showing any symptoms as their

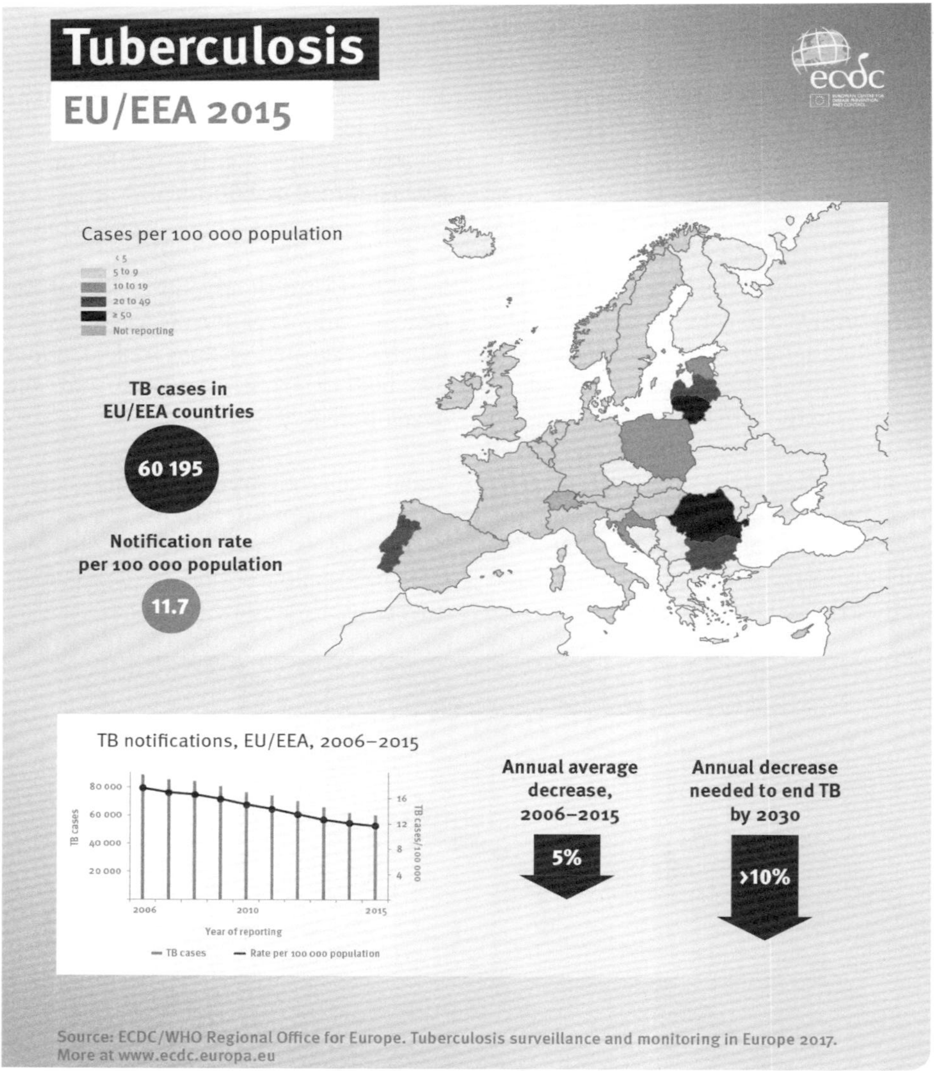

▲ *(2) Overview of tuberculosis in Europe by the ECDC*

immune system is strong enough to keep the bacteria wrapped-up in the lung tissue. Secondly, patients with active tuberculosis show the following symptoms: coughing (blood), chest pain, unintentional loss of weight, chills, fever etc.

In addition, the expert also informed about the new webpage dzk-tuberkulose.de, which is newly developed to inform people about the disease and about the chances to fight against it.

What, on the other hand, are the symptoms of bovine tuberculosis in the animals? DVM Fischer-Tenhagen of the Free University broadened the minds not only of the medical students, but impressed the audience with her expertise on bovine tuberculosis. In her passionate talk, she explained the spread and the undertaken control measurements in Germany and diagnostic methods in the veterinary clinic. Many affected cows do not show any symptoms, which is named asymptomatic. In symptomatic individuals, the disease can cause a slight fever, the lymph nodes swell and the cows are coughing and appear weak. Next to symptoms which are linked to the respiratory system, the mycobacteria can infect the digestive system and may result in diarrhoea and constipation. Furthermore, the diagnostic is challenging and next to well-known tests with tuberculin, Fischer-Tenhagen referred to another diagnostic method: the so-called Hero- Rats. These rats are trained to identify positive samples and show a high sensitivity and specificity.

How relevant is tuberculosis nowadays? Professor Dr. Timo Ulrichs, Head of Department International Emergency and Disaster Relief and Global Health at the Akkon University for Human Science, gave a talk about tuberculosis as a worldwide problem for humans and about the infection itself. He reminded the audience about the 9.6 million new cases (source from the year 2014) and the actual relevance of this nearly forgotten sickness. For sure, it is more relevant for the less wealthy countries, according to Prof. Ulrichs, but because of the globalisation process it is an issue the whole world needs to be aware of.

Furthermore, with the new rise of tuberculosis in Eastern European countries, the disease may be associated with refugees. People leaving their countries because of civil wars face many challenges and a long way to safer places. Under these extreme circumstances their health and immune defence suffers and they are at a higher risk contracting infectious diseases.

Finally, the audience gained insights on the relevance of tuberculosis for societies relying on pastoralism. Antonia Braus from Vétérinaires Sans Frontières e.V. Germany gave an insight on how animal health is becoming increasingly important, especially to people in the pastoral communities, as their lives directly depend on their animals. In addition, she explained some challenges that tuberculosis presents, such as the difficulty of differentiating types of bacteria. Through insufficient hygiene measures, bacteria from the gastrointestinal tract can reach the outer genital organs and can induce an atypical infection of the urogenital tract, leaving the tuberculosis undiagnosed. Braus stressed the importance of educating and raising awareness around proper hygiene and prevention measures. She also mentioned the need for more research on zoonosis, e.g.

All speakers of this event agreed on a collaborative approach to tackle this global challenge. Cooperatively with the expert DVM Baumann, Head of the FAO Reference Centre for Veterinary Public Health, Prof. DVM Doherr of the Faculty of Veterinary Medicine of the Free University Berlin gave the guests an insight into the concept and the veterinarian contribution to the One Health principles. Firstly, the guests were given a general overview of the One Health approach and its national and global development in the last years. They outlined that veterinarians still need to be taken more into consideration for Public Health guidelines and highlighted that veterinary skills are crucial to tackle Global Health challenges, e.g. control and prevention of outbreaks and especially zoonosis.

After a break with snacks, drinks, and friendly conversation, the evening resumed with the interactive part of the workshop: The World Café.

The participants divided into groups and visited separate tables, each held by one expert, to exchange opinions and discuss the various topics.

With a total of five tables and individual themes, each group got to visit three before the plenum reunited to gather their final thoughts.

At the first table, participants reflected on the concept of One Health. They discussed the importance of collaboration and the presence of intergovernmental organisations such as the World Organisation for Animal Health (OiE) and the World Health Organization (WHO). However, some believed this might not be enough, as there is little to no direct contact with national governments, that are far more impactful locally. Some wondered, within Germany, do we need a Federal Ministry to promote and further the One Health movement? Globalisation was also discussed, especially the influence it can have on diseases. For instance, as large migration movements have been entering Europe in recent years, Eastern European countries have witnessed a new rise of tuberculosis. How can we solve this problem without discouraging globalisation? Most emphasis, participants agreed, should be placed on creating a prominent dialogue.

Next, bovine tuberculosis and diagnostic procedures were discussed at the second table. Participants agreed that a highly sensitive, primary screening would be best to minimize patients that go undiagnosed. A second screening to examine patients more closely could follow. Most essential is the applicability of the procedure, especially when imagining is used in newly industrialised and developing countries. It must be mobile and cost efficient. Before such procedures are realised, it is crucial to educate and raise awareness around safe and clean handling of animals. Tuberculosis can be considered as a poverty associated disease.

At the third table, participants discussed this correlation using examples learned in the previous presentations. Antimicrobial resistance is more prevalent in Asian countries, where awareness about the correct usage of antibiotics is lacking. What are further explanations for the rising numbers of tuberculosis cases next to poverty? For instance, an HIV infection can enhance the mechanisms of a tuberculosis infection. "Needle sharing" is the most frequent cause for HIV in the Ukraine, proving once more the importance of awareness around hygiene in countries across the map. To achieve a higher level of awareness, and better disease prevention, a strategy needs to be developed. For achieving this, a participant noted, we need to reconcile academia and society, remain pragmatic and realistic.

At the fourth table, participants tackled the broad topic of zoonosis. A student summarised the main issue with a simple sketch on the board. She drew a line as a time axis, wrote animals on the left end, humans on the right, and marked the middle. She then explained that diagnostic procedures are only applied once a zoonosis has clinically appeared in human patients and drew an arrow to the right of the middle mark. Our goal would be to shift the arrow to the left, meaning that we should work on detecting zoonosis before they reach humans, studying the animals more carefully.

Here, it would perhaps be useful to have more organisational collaboration. The Food and Agriculture Organization (FAO) sometimes serves as a halfway point between the OiE, associated with animals, and the WHO, associated with humans. However, participants felt that no organisation fully bridges the gap and that this is especially needed to deal with the issue of zoonosis. Public services could be of help, along with further research in epidemiology and the development of vaccines.

Finally, to provide some cultural and societal insight, participants at the fifth table learned more about pastoralism. Vétérinaires Sans Frontières e.V. Germany has a long tradition of working with pastoralists in Eastern Africa, and are caring for the animal health and food security of the herds. Participants at the VSF table were talking about cheap and effective ways of preventing diseases like brucellosis and tuberculosis to be spread. They also dived into political issues as they were discussing the role of women in pastoral societies and how strengthening their influence in economic matters can lead to more advanced and thus safer milk production.

Lively discussions and new ideas were held and exchanged at all tables, which results were summarised and presented by a student from each group in the end.

All participants and experts together then drafted demands to politicians and universities, named in the following:

- stronger cooperation between the three Global Health leaders - WHO, FAO and OIE - as well as national organisations and ministries
- more funding into One Health research
- more education of the public about zoonosis
- better connection between universities and study fields, through tandems or shared courses.

A very informative, eye-opening and exciting evening ended. Everyone came together once more for a drink and a snack, and many contact details were exchanged. Highly motivated and full of new ideas, the participants of the transdisciplinary workshop finished the evening and were already promising their return for next year's event!

Sources and Notes:
(1] "One Health: A New Professional Imperative" (PDF). American Veterinary Medical Association. 15 July 2008. Retrieved 2017-11-23.
(2) Source: ECDC/WHO Regional Office of Europe. Tuberculosis surveillance and monitoring in Europe 2017. More at www.ecdc.europa.eu. Retrieved 2017-11-26.
(3) Funded by Engagement Global with financial support of the Federal Ministry of Economic Cooperation and Development. The editor is responsible for the content of this publication; the described positions do not represent the perspective of Engagement Global gGmbH and the Federal Ministry of Economic Cooperation and Development.

3. Humanitarian Congress 2017

Regina Felicitas Clemenz

The XIX. Humanitarian Congress 2017 under the motto "Out of order? Reshaping humanitarism" was taking place in the university campus of the Charité in Berlin. The event was frequently visited by a very international audience of about 800 people over the weekend of the 13th to the 14th of October. It brought together a wide range of multi discipliner experts from the field, medical, humanitarian and international organisations, offered politicians to take part and share their views. Also including the media as well as young professionals interested in the humanitarian sector. The general aim is to create a platform to connect, share experiences and expertise, discuss and find an approach to handle the future of sometimes overwhelming complex problems due to climate change, political issues, protracted emergencies and security problems.

As it is for a single person impossible to visit all of the keynote speeches, panel discussions and workshops at the same time, I can only give a review about the ones which I attended. It was criticised by a lot of visitors in the closing remarks that the topics and the way of reporting would have been repetitive over the recent years of the event and there was the demand for a more critical point of view towards recent political developments. Especially the refugee crisis in the Mediterranean where migrants are now mainly stuck in inhumane conditions in EU-sponsored detention centres and access is denied to humanitarian workers was controversially discussed. But for newly involved participants like me the given informations were still valuable and the exchange with such a international society of same minded workers from the humanitarian field is at least a open door to possibilities. How this is used depends on every individual itself.

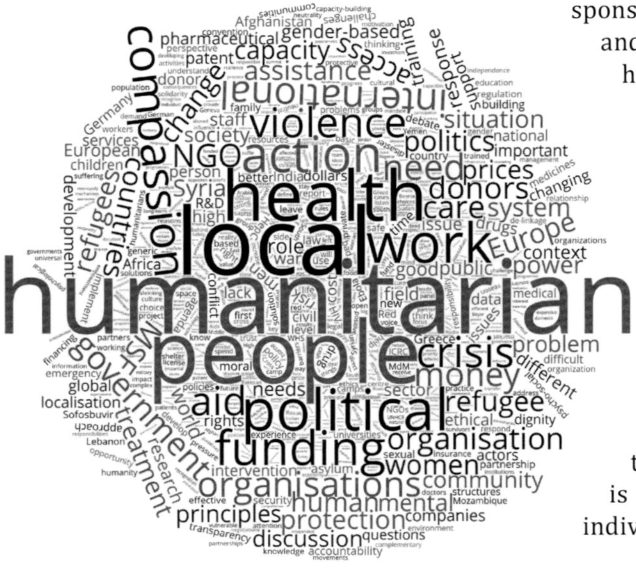

The programme was addressing the following topics:

- adapting to a changing political landscape
- Yemen: a never ending war
- contribution of humanitarians to IHL compliance
- CHS & measuring success in humanitarian interventions
- negotiating with non-state actors
- sexual & reproductive health: safe abortion care
- an introduction to medical humanitarian aid
- refugees and migrants in northern africa
- humanitarianism: an anthropological perpective
- mainstreaming community based disaster risk management in fragile and conflict sensitive context
- criminalisation of humanitarian aid
- news in humanitarian aid
- global surgery
- The return of famine?
- palliative care
- scientific session
- snakebites – a multifacted fatal neglect
- humanitarian aid and development
- local partners in emergencies and cluster system
- Q&A: becoming a humanitarian aid worker
- film screening: Minutes to Die, Snakebite: The World's Ignored Health Crisis
- closing remarks

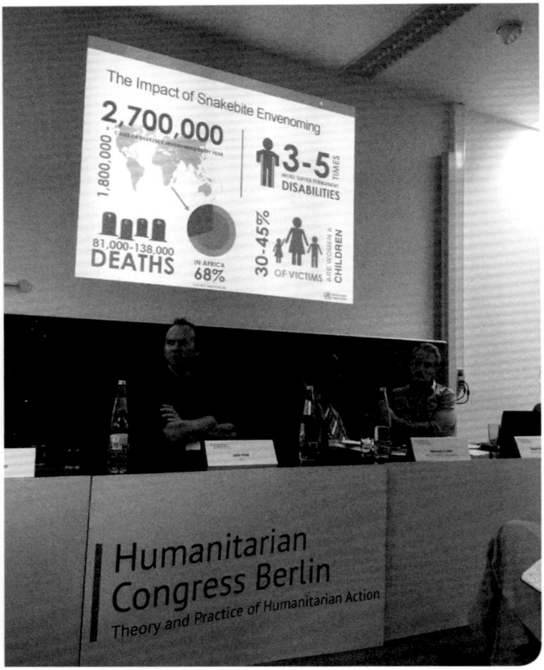

▲ *The Impact of Snakebite Envenoming*
Source: WHO 2017

While records of the events in the main room are available on Youtube and linked on the official website of the Humanitarian Congress for further access, unfortunately the sessions held in the smaller rooms are not recorded and abstracts or reports about this congress are hard to find, so I'd like to give an impression of an outstanding panel discussion.

The session with the title "Snakebite, a multifaceted fatal neglect" was probably the most eye opening report among the others and therefore should be mentioned in this publication. The panel was hosting Mr. Abdulrazaq G. Habib (Professor and Consultant Physician, Department of Medicine, Bayero University, Kano, Nigeria), Mrs. Bernadette Abela-Ridder (Team Leader, Neglected Zoonotic Diseases, WHO Department of Control of Neglected Tropical Diseases), Mr. Julien Potet (Neglected Tropical Disease Policy Advisor, MSF Access Campaign) an the german politician Mrs. Kordula Schulz-Asche (Member of the German Bundestag, Alliance 90/The Green Party) under the chair of Mr. Benjamin Waldmann (Programme Manager for Snakebite, Health Action International (HAI)).

In the report and the visually even more highlighting following film screening with the title "Snakebites, minutes to die" it was illustrated impressively how poverty, suffering, disabilities and deaths of specifically this Neglected Tropical Disease are a nature related crisis going hand in hand with a man made one. Especially the shared experience of a snakebite surviver who was among the audiences and the extensive report of Mr. Habib who also did a lot of assessment in the field expressed in combination with the database how less the humanitarian sector is equipped to respond to this need. It was compelling to follow the performance and the take home message was without any doubt that if there was an international awareness and approach but especially a political will which would reach beyond the borders of well set up countries, so much avoidable damage to individuals, society and economy could be prevented with relatively easy and inexpensive actions.

It might be surprising that in a lot of rural development areas snakebites are more or at least equally feared as HIV, TBC and Malaria. The worldwide distribution of incidences is variable and the venomous snakebites that occur each year may be depending on the source as many as five million, but they could result in about 2.5 million poisonings and 20,000 to 125,000 deaths, not covering the numbers of disabilities, severe infections and other medical complications. Snakebites are mainly not paid attention to due to being a non communicable disease and they hit mainly the poorest and least empowered people who are exposed under their simple living conditions to this threat. Up to 45% are women and children living in rural areas, working on farms and already at or below the poverty line are affected.

In many countries, most dramatically in India, the government makes no effort to do proper assessment or evaluation, the existing statistics are mostly non governmental and definitely incomplete, with estimating a degree of under-reporting of over 70% worldwide, especially in rural or weak infrastructure equipped areas. The lack of verified statistics may therefore also play a huge role why the international support for areas of high incidences is nearly inexistent. Nevertheless it was stressed frequently that it is also a matter of ignorance rather than simply missing information. This applies both to the pharmaceutical industry where the only supplier of antivenoms for half the continent of Africa was cutting of production by 100% without giving any alternatives or any other company addressing the supply gap same as of the ministries of health in charge for the affected countries.

As the population in especially African countries know that they have less support to expect from official health facilities which are only exceptionally not under equipped, untrained and out of stock for antivenoms, help is sought primarily in traditional healers which are affordable for the victims. If professional support is even attended it is often too late as the timeframe for the treatment depending on the snake species may be very short. As a result of insufficient knowledge, exorbitantly high fees for medical care, a lack of trust in medicine and simply not accessible or existing health facilities the consequences are the loss of a limb, permanent disabilities, psychological distress or even death.

The impact of snakebite related damage to not only the individual but society and also economy of the affected countries must be immense, but remains a matter of speculations. While South American countries are despite their general medical set up having an affordable or even free treatment program for their population, other development countries in Africa and Asia are far from these options. So it is not surprising that the incident of a snakebite is putting years of being in debts as a burden on the remaining family members what will also contradict any kind of development. Even more drastically it exposes women whose husband passed away in restrictive religious and traditional areas to extreme poverty, bitten girls who might have survived but stay physical and psychological battered won't have the chance to get married and will therefore be even more vulnerable. But who ever was bitten, a stigmatisation is nearly certainly an additional social burden apart from the challenges of everyday life.

Humanitarian Congress Berlin

Theory and Practice of Humanitarian Action

Even that the effects of the neglect are outcrying, approaches of global players like the WHO remain insufficient and snakebite stays largely unfunded and ignored among global public health priorities and have not been subject to substantial control programs by the international community. Despite this according to Mrs. Abela-Ridder it has to be seen as a small win that snakebite is listed since 2017 by the WHO among other Neglected Tropical Diseases again and not like in previous years just under a sub-definition of "Other neglected conditions" wich are hardly getting any attention. Even if snakebites would be without the massive under reporting probably leading the list of incidences and deaths of NTDs, there are just few research attempts. The speech highlighted therefore that global healthcare is very politicised and the actual need and damage is not automatically related to a linear amount of funding, approach and awareness.

This health crisis is a master example for how capitalism in addition to monopolistic suppliers are taking a huge toll on populations unless good governance or at least action of the global public health authorities are addressing the problems.The outlook to the future shows unfortunately that there will presumably remain a huge gap of education, both for medical staff and the population itself which are due to the lack of save and affordable medication available the only prevention measurements and there is no major change to hope for in the next years, probably also not from the WHO. Even though their logo contains ironically a snake.

But in the agenda of the SDG's there has to be a change in global thinking: if development is wanted to be achieved, education and medical care are among other needs the base and congresses like this one offering the opportunity to discuss these urgent themes while involving as many parties as possible.

4. World Health Summit 2017 Reports on different workshops and sessions

Gaby Feldmann, Delia Grün, Hannah Sendler

4.1 Introduction

The World Health Summit, held annually during October in Berlin, is considered one of the most important international forums for global health issues, strategic developments and health decisions.

The summit began in 2009 on the occasion of the 300th year anniversary of the Charité – Universitätsmedizin Berlin. The founders recognized that whilst similar gatherings of leaders were well established in fields such as economic development and technology, a global forum did not exist for medical practice, research and health care systems.

From October 15 to 17, 2017, the eighth World Health Summit brought together 2,000 political, scientific, business and civil society representatives from nearly 100 countries to discuss current global health care issues.

Those to ask this year are: How to fight antibiotic resistance, how high-tech medicine can be affordable and what needs to be done to improve health care systems?

International, interdisciplinary and academically independent – the World Health Summit is the exemplary platform to showcase the immense challenges of and the latest developments in international healthcare and the latest developments in international healthcare, as well as to jointly develop strategies to tackle these major health care issues work together on solutions.

The summit is still under the patronage of the German chancellor, President of the French Republic, and the President of the European Commission (World Health Summit, Berlin, Germany, October 15–17, 2017, Program).

As participants of this unique event, we will give an overview of the most important contributions on the following pages.

WORLD
HEALTH
SUMMIT

4.2 Workshop/Sessions

4.2.1 Governing the Future with the Sustainable Development Goals

Keynote 05

"The 2030 Agenda for Sustainable Development aims to shape a very different world. The factors that now govern the wellbeing of the human condition, and the planet that sustains it, are no longer so discrete. Health plays a central role in this challenging agenda as a precondition, outcome, and indicator of a sustainable society. The SDGs recognize that health challenges can no longer be addressed by the health sector acting alone – nearly everyone of the SDGs can contribute to improving health and wellbeing. The SDGs also underline that governments will need the support of many other stakeholders to address the determinants of health and priority health issues such as NCDs, UHC and poverty related diseases."

(World Health Summit, Berlin, Germany, October 15–17, 2017, Program, P. 126)

Introduction

Chair Ilona Kickbusch, The Graduate Institute of International and Development Studies, Global Health Center, Director, Switzerland

The 2030 Agenda for Sustainable Development Goals (SDGs)

- The Sustainable Development Goals (SDGs) are a universal call to action to end poverty, protect the planet and ensure that all people enjoy peace and prosperity.

- The adoption of the 17 SDGs marks the first time, that the international community agreed on an universal catalogue of fixed time-specific targets covering all three dimensions of sustainability – social, environment, economy. These targets will play a key role in international cooperation in core policy fields in the next decades.

- The objective of the 2030 Agenda for Sustainable Development is to make global development sustainable on a social, ecological and economic level and in doing so substantially boost the long overdue transformation of global economies towards a much more sustainable and inclusive development.

Criticizing the Sustainable Development Goals is clear at the following points

+ It is a comprehensive set of indicators.

+ It creates a close connection to administrative statistics and political processes.

- The validity of the headline indicators and the reliability of the individual indicators are questionable.

- The design based on the "EU Sustainable Development Strategy" (SDS) and a lack of integrated overall concept make information sources diffuse.

- It is non-binding in the implementation.

- It recurs mainly on technical and governmental challenges.

- Only one goal deals with health, but health is the core.

- Health is both: output and input.

Given the significant political, economic and social changes that the world has seen, when the Sustainable Development Goals were adopted, they are facing some old new challenges:

■ Warlike disputes and economic hardship drove migration to record high

■ Dramatic political contexts

■ Strong commercial drivers (e.g. food and tobacco industry)

"Current challenges and opportunities for accelerating progress on the Health SDGs in 2030"

Nancy Fulman, Institute for Health Metrics and Evaluation, Scientific Advisor

New health data and current challenges

- "Intersectoral action is vital to achieving faster health gains":
  - Worldwide the total number of road traffic deaths has plateaued at 1.25 million per year, with the highest road traffic fatality rates in low-income countries. While there has been progress towards improving road safety legislation and in making vehicles safer, urgent action is needed.
- "Substantial acceleration of progress is required in the SDG era":
  - Child overweight projections show rising prevalence – unless action is taken.
  - Childhood overweight and obesity have increased dramatically since 1990. They are associated with serious health problems and the risk of premature illness and death later in life.
- "Lowest scores on the health-related SDG-index in 2016: Yet vaccine coverage scores are high for many countries":
  - Country performance for the health-related SDG index varied in 2016, underscoring health inequalities across and within countries. Afghanistan, the Central African Republic and Somalia rank the lowest on the index.

	SDG index	MDG index	Non-MDG index	Disaster mort	Child stunting	Child wasting	Child overweight	MMR	SBA	Under-5 mort	NN mort	HIV incid	Tuberculosis incid	Malaria incid	Hep B incid	NTD prev	NCD mort	Suicide mort	Alcohol use	Road injury mort	FP need met, mod	Adol birth rate	UHC index	Air poll mort	WaSH mort	Poisoning mort	Smoking prev	Vaccine cov	Int partner viol	Water	Sanitation	Hygiene	HH air poll	Occ burden	Mean $PM_{2.5}$	Homicide	Conflict mort	Violence prev	Child sex abuse	Cert death reg
1 Singapore	87	91	84	100	96	85	59	89	100	100	100	54	63	100	87	100	90	53	88	98	80	94	95	74	78	100	86	95	99	96	99	97	100	74	50	99	100	97	42	100
2 Iceland	86	96	79	100	100	99	32	100	100	100	100	60	86	100	100	100	94	43	56	95	94	88	100	98	93	85	63	90	98	100	100	100	100	68	91	95	100	94	47	95
3 Sweden	86	95	81	100	100	98	53	98	100	97	95	62	93	100	100	100	94	38	40	99	88	84	98	100	85	68	77	96	95	100	99	100	99	88	100	84	100	75	29	90
4 Norway	84	95	80	56	100	99	53	98	100	96	92	63	96	100	100	100	92	47	54	98	90	82	99	97	83	87	61	93	98	100	100	100	100	86	88	93	100	94	52	88
5 Netherlands	83	94	79	100	100	99	67	89	100	88	80	66	98	100	98	100	86	49	49	94	92	95	97	82	87	100	54	86	98	100	100	100	100	70	66	90	100	82	39	89
6 Finland	83	97	78	100	100	98	64	99	100	100	98	71	98	100	100	100	92	32	22	94	98	80	100	100	100	85	53	96	97	100	100	100	100	91	96	77	100	84	50	100
7 Israel	82	90	78	100	99	98	48	90	99	90	88	58	100	100	92	100	92	57	84	70	84	72	87	84	80	89	53	93	87	99	98	99	100	97	59	68	72	84	24	84
8 Malta	81	85	77	70	100	98	25	91	99	77	63	49	95	100	97	100	88	77	64	99	76	54	88	81	96	97	51	93	96	100	99	100	100	76	74	83	100	98	44	96
9 Switzerland	80	94	75	55	100	98	61	92	100	88	77	56	95	100	70	100	98	40	44	98	93	100	100	96	96	100	44	85	99	100	100	100	100	66	78	94	100	94	43	92
10 UK	80	89	77	89	97	99	53	86	99	84	78	55	84	100	96	100	82	56	39	97	98	62	88	82	86	84	44	93	97	100	100	100	100	73	75	97	100	91	36	96
11 Australia	80	91	75	77	96	98	54	92	99	88	82	63	100	100	74	100	94	44	23	79	100	62	96	100	90	85	64	94	98	96	99	97	100	78	96	80	100	94	47	96
12 Canada	79	89	74	100	98	99	47	84	99	80	72	57	100	100	82	100	87	43	36	74	94	68	92	98	83	75	65	60	97	100	97	100	100	61	90	76	100	94	41	96
13 Germany	78	92	73	100	100	99	54	83	99	90	86	60	94	100	98	100	81	44	34	89	91	80	92	82	87	100	38	74	100	100	99	100	100	71	70	93	100	91	34	90
14 Italy	78	92	70	49	100	98	35	97	99	93	86	54	96	100	79	100	91	69	38	69	81	84	94	87	100	96	43	93	98	98	99	99	100	76	65	93	100	90	44	94
15 Denmark	77	93	71	100	100	99	44	96	99	87	79	61	95	100	97	100	82	46	21	93	90	92	92	86	84	90	51	91	98	100	100	100	100	54	79	91	100	83	51	90
16 Belgium	77	91	73	100	100	98	69	87	99	88	84	54	90	100	93	100	82	27	34	70	91	75	93	79	83	83	46	96	96	100	100	100	100	71	64	80	62	83	44	85
17 Antigua and Barbuda	76	69	79	100	89	91	44	55	99	64	57	53	83	100	84	97	65	100	79	67	91	37	61	77	59	63	100	100	84	63	80	77	99	87	66	46	100	92	75	79
18 Cyprus	76	91	70	85	100	98	45	80	99	92	88	55	88	100	92	100	83	77	46	58	90	86	89	75	87	96	26	94	95	100	99	100	100	72	60	71	100	99	44	70
19 Slovenia	75	91	69	59	89	84	40	88	100	99	92	93	93	100	93	100	82	27	37	80	67	98	93	77	96	77	35	95	98	88	95	99	97	69	60	87	100	100	73	92
20 Ireland	75	91	69	100	100	98	46	92	100	88	81	54	93	100	89	100	86	46	11	90	91	73	93	87	94	77	44	90	98	100	99	100	100	86	83	93	100	93	33	98
21 Japan	75	93	69	19	95	95	81	90	99	97	100	78	83	100	75	100	100	24	61	94	66	93	98	97	82	74	32	96	100	96	99	97	100	69	71	99	100	95	39	88
22 Austria	74	93	69	54	100	98	64	98	100	91	86	54	92	100	100	100	86	37	24	87	92	80	96	83	100	82	25	88	100	100	98	100	100	80	66	94	100	100	44	95
23 Spain	74	92	67	100	100	96	36	92	94	92	88	51	89	100	94	100	92	67	10	89	87	75	98	94	97	94	25	97	100	100	100	100	100	98	80	97	100	100	49	91
24 USA	74	83	72	58	98	100	58	60	99	75	67	51	100	100	88	100	70	36	41	51	83	54	79	82	84	56	68	88	96	100	96	100	100	77	83	43	100	100	37	94
25 Brunei	74	76	74	66	86	87	69	56	99	68	64	49	53	100	67	100	59	76	99	47	83	49	65	90	77	63	68	97	88	96	98	97	100	30	95	80	100	91	42	86
26 France	73	92	68	82	100	98	64	85	100	88	84	64	92	100	99	100	86	29	20	78	95	72	94	98	87	83	28	90	97	100	99	100	100	63	74	88	100	82	74	84
27 Barbados	73	68	77	100	89	75	62	46	99	58	43	46	83	100	80	100	64	75	53	60	90	40	61	77	59	78	97	83	85	75	81	78	100	93	61	31	100	90	75	85
28 South Korea	72	90	65	73	96	94	40	78	100	90	92	74	50	80	74	98	89	9	55	51	91	100	95	77	80	60	46	98	94	96	99	97	100	79	44	77	100	91	42	88
29 Czech Republic	72	89	67	86	97	87	55	90	100	96	94	85	98	100	88	100	68	40	21	74	68	72	86	64	80	79	29	98	95	88	96	99	99	63	58	83	100	93	70	92
30 Slovakia	72	83	70	68	89	85	60	86	100	78	74	95	93	100	89	100	56	44	26	70	72	51	75	56	88	68	44	98	89	88	95	99	99	81	56	66	100	87	74	97
31 Taiwan (Province of China)	72	86	66	37	93	94	45	73	98	84	82	77	71	100	51	77	74	34	66	46	100	82	79	67	79	67	68	98	82	82	94	95	98	70	44	76	100	86	85	88
32 New Zealand	71	86	66	37	96	98	39	76	100	80	73	66	95	100	86	100	86	42	29	72	95	48	89	100	86	82	54	91	92	96	98	97	100	63	100	80	100	73	2	100
33 Poland	71	82	68	100	88	84	61	94	100	85	77	80	82	100	97	100	58	31	35	61	50	62	78	58	90	83	28	96	95	87	94	99	97	71	48	74	100	100	70	78
34 Estonia	70	85	65	100	91	91	52	92	100	93	95	59	75	100	81	100	61	28	10	77	82	69	83	80	97	59	37	93	93	85	82	97	94	89	98	48	100	98	30	99
35 Portugal	70	87	64	68	99	98	41	79	100	93	91	32	76	100	84	99	84	47	9	67	86	73	87	88	86	79	47	92	95	99	95	99	99	78	82	79	100	92	44	85
36 Costa Rica	70	75	66	46	90	90	29	59	99	65	53	57	86	100	71	64	94	62	56	46	96	29	73	82	67	77	87	96	75	88	96	80	97	93	59	37	100	82	16	97
37 Luxembourg	70	94	62	100	100	99	45	80	99	100	100	52	92	100	98	100	90	49	2	85	95	85	98	83	89	94	43	97	99	100	100	100	100	84	64	87	100	96	44	86
38 Cuba	70	72	69	40	86	91	56	52	99	81	80	39	95	100	90	73	65	39	58	71	98	31	70	68	60	79	59	95	86	67	80	82	99	60	63	46	100	92	74	98
39 Mauritius	69	67	70	53	83	43	44	48	99	58	45	62	73	100	58	94	49	54	72	58	82	43	66	67	66	91	53	98	71	72	96	98	99	78	68	63	100	86	70	91
40 Maldives	69	67	71	66	64	50	78	49	98	73	62	93	56	100	65	100	78	85	92	64	78	92	79	56	64	100	36	95	63	36	81	72	97	77	47	84	100	87	70	63
41 Greece	68	89	61	100	100	98	35	82	99	88	82	62	100	100	68	100	80	86	32	57	65	78	90	76	100	81	4	81	96	100	99	100	100	82	76	86	100	91	44	77
42 Croatia	68	83	64	100	88	84	46	82	100	85	76	91	85	100	88	100	59	32	31	64	52	72	79	56	92	91	10	95	96	86	95	99	95	71	57	80	100	97	73	93
43 Albania	68	65	69	100	61	56	26	81	99	59	50	100	82	100	84	100	64	69	55	70	17	45	69	48	86	64	52	100	85	73	83	95	83	59	67	65	100	95	79	62
44 Seychelles	68	66	68	100	85	79	55	59	97	63	48	51	64	100	50	39	51	53	68	48	87	25	56	67	60	55	62	100	59	70	88	95	99	67	69	42	100	80	70	83
45 Uruguay	67	74	65	100	85	94	33	63	99	69	63	46	74	100	84	99	60	25	49	43	78	24	65	78	70	66	38	96	83	94	98	96	99	56	75	46	100	85	53	83
46 Hungary	67	82	63	100	96	93	51	76	99	80	74	88	91	100	90	100	43	21	22	73	67	54	75	49	79	78	20	98	91	87	91	99	94	68	50	74	100	88	73	99
47 Panama	67	62	71	40	72	95	71	43	93	54	50	37	60	60	73	89	85	68	55	45	94	21	62	75	54	62	100	74	76	79	76	85	93	91	68	20	100	94	66	92
48 Mexico	67	67	68	52	79	91	58	50	98	56	50	52	73	84	71	78	74	68	54	42	87	22	57	69	58	60	73	76	82	88	88	85	94	74	58	18	100	100	79	92
49 The Bahamas	66	68	67	18	89	91	60	45	99	65	60	37	60	100	79	100	51	94	60	44	92	38	58	72	60	74	94	96	76	69	84	81	98	94	72	14	100	86	74	80
50 Grenada	66	65	67	51	86	90	53	57	99	57	43	55	86	100	79	72	37	60	51	44	87	46	47	57	52	54	85	98	74	62	73	78	98	80	61	39	100	88	74	87
51 Colombia	66	68	66	40	82	96	83	47	97	56	44	54	72	45	73	51	88	69	50	46	96	32	66	65	64	80	77	94	62	80	92	79	92	99	62	2	100	67	66	94
52 Malaysia	66	72	61	90	69	51	34	50	99	78	75	63	53	82	52	34	58	53	86	30	84	59	65	52	61	48	47	97	66	78	96	97	100	60	61	70	100	86	60	54
53 Saint Lucia	65	64	68	30	96	88	84	39	98	54	35	61	67	100	85	58	59	60	49	46	86	35	56	75	61	84	79	98	74	62	80	82	98	94	62	20	100	85	75	88
54 Jamaica	65	59	69	61	90	92	70	51	98	50	38	43	87	100	78	67	54	95	58	63	85	19	59	66	55	70	78	96	72	59	58	58	94	68	66	10	100	90	67	79
55 Jordan	65	73	64	100	87	85	77	56	100	54	41	100	91	100	61	77	62	89	96	41	59	50	67	57	70	52	31	99	36	81	96	88	100	100	36	54	10	64	76	72
56 Trinidad and Tobago	65	64	68	68	99	82	67	44	99	50	30	46	78	100	75	96	46	39	71	41	76	52	54	66	59	76	62	54	77	65	84	79	100	94	62	14	100	86	74	96
57 Armenia	65	69	63	44	71	82	37	69	99	62	55	72	63	100	63	99	50	59	61	68	40	46	65	46	78	48	34	94	84	87	77	89	91	54	47	55	100	91	100	98

▲ *"Highest scores on the health-related SDG-index in 2016: Child overweight, suicide mortality, alcohol use among main challenges"*

Source: http://www.thelancet.com/pdfs/journals/lancet/PIIS0140-6736(17)32336-X.pdf

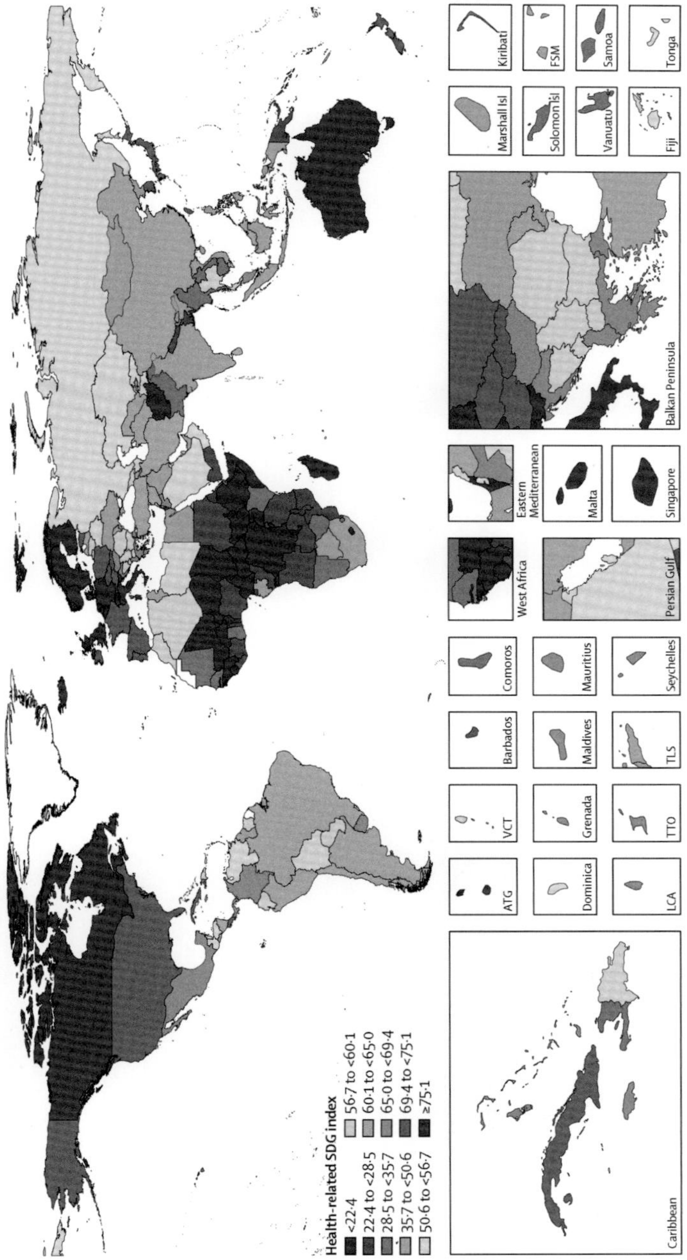

▲ *"Mapping the health-related SDG Index in 2016:*
Large geographically inequalities to overcome in the next 13 years"

Source: http://www.thelancet.com/pdfs/journals/lancet/PIIS0140-6736(17)32336-X.pdf

Key Messages

- The rallying cry of the Sustainable Development Goals is to 'leave no one behind' by 2030 – and to reach those who are furthest behind first.
- Additional financing is needed to realize this promise, particularly in the poorest countries.
- Health should be given priority among the three core elements of a basic social compact – social protection, education and basic universal healthcare.
- Every country has its own story. A very surprising thing is the high maternal mortality in the United States.

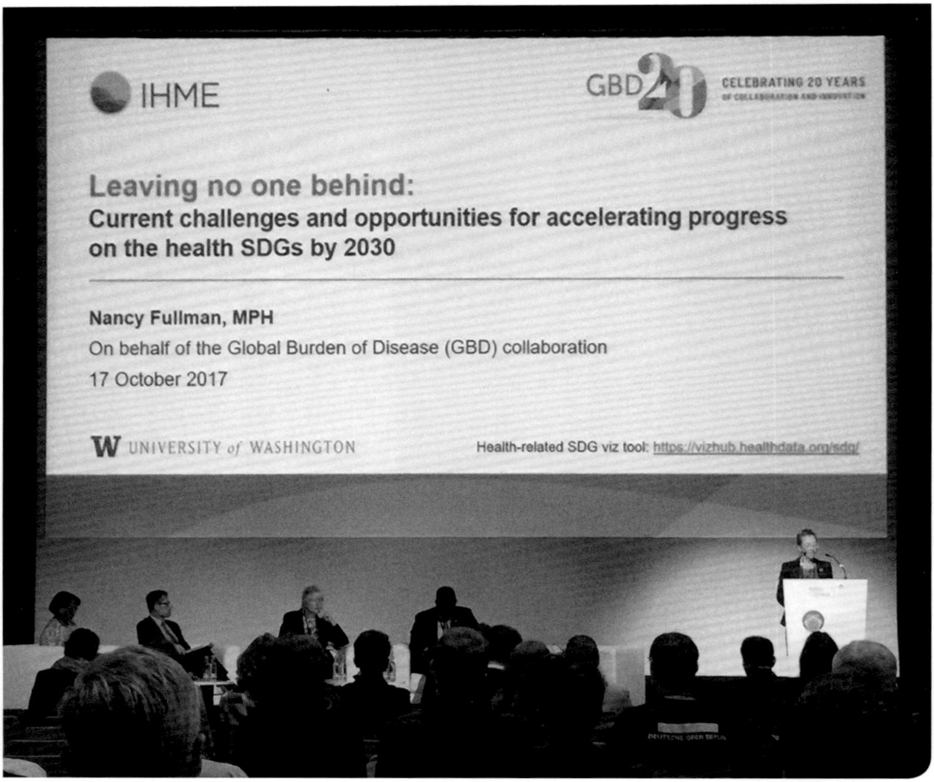

▲ *"Leaving no one behind": that's the Key Message of the Speakers Nancy Fulman, Dr. Matshidiso Rebecca Moeti, Justin McCarthy, Elhadj As Sy and Chair Ilona Kickbusch.*

"How is WHO and WHO/Africa in particular approaching the intersectoral approach to the SDGs? Will the WHO work differently?"

Matshidiso Rebecca Moeti, World Health organization (WHO), WHO Regional Office for Africa, Regional Director for Africa, Congo

Key Messages

- The focus of public health interventions is to prevent and manage diseases, injuries and other health conditions through surveillance of cases and the promotion of healthy behavior, communities, and environments.

- Health as "political issue".

- Demand for more financial help requires underlining the economic advantages to get support from politics.

- Interaction with the commercial sector has been broadened and deepened. Entrepreneurial involvement can serve as a catalyst for economic and social development.

- The tasks of WHO must be responsive to the needs of a country or region. "Transfer of framework" to all countries could be useful.

- "Learning from management processes" in other fields is a goal for WHO in future.

"What Changes for the Private Sector? Does it live up to its Global Responsibilities in the SDG Context? Especially in Health?"

Justin McCarthy, Pfizer Inc.,Global Policy and International Affairs, Senior Vice President, United States of America

Key Messages

- Goal 17 (Revitalize the global partnership for sustainable development) is critical: shift from pure charity to what?

- Need of more sustainable partnerships; offer of "cooperation with other partners"

- Good example: Gavi, the Vaccine Alliance: It is a public–private global health partnership committed to increasing access to immunisation in poor countries. It brings together developing country and donor governments, WHO, UNICEF, World Bank, the vaccine industry in both industrialised and developing countries, research and technical agencies, civil society, the Bill & Melinda Gates Foundation and other private philanthropists.

- Commitment to long-term responsibility

"Can the SDGs Really Help Address the Many Disasters and Emergencies we are Facing?"

Elhadj As Sy, International Federation of the Red Cross (IFRC), Secretary General, Switzerland

Key Messages

- The number of geophysical and natural disasters taking place each year is skyrocketing. Since 1970, the number of disasters worldwide has more than quadrupled to around 400 a year.

- Disasters and climate related catastrophes are increasing the dangers facing children today such as child trafficking.

- Protection of the humanitarian space for the health workers is one of the most important challenges in the future.

- The range of actors involved in driving capacity development and implementing programmes is broad and encompasses several different groups. The emergency preparedness for response and recovery from disasters by strengthening local actors must be ensured.

- Early action is vital. It is necessary to build early partnerships, not until the disasters have occured.

- It is important to ensure that health is not isolated. It is not something "by the way" or "on top of it".

SUMMING-UP

by Chair Ilona Kickbusch

- Numerous exemplary initiatives give courage and hope.
- Around the world, amid widespread progress, many people remain marginalised, extremely poor and ill.
- These inequalities can be overlooked when progress is measured in averages across the whole population, as was the case with the Sustainable Development Goals (SDGs).
- Understanding where there are gaps, and taking early and sustained action to address them is critical if we are to translate this ambitious "leave no one behind" commitment into action.
- Leadership is the key to fulfilling the Sustainable Development Goals (SDGs). But not in the narrow outlook of power, status and authority. Local leaders, the people who care deeply about community issues, who implement initiatives and who shape local development, represent a huge window of opportunity for global social change.
- Good things come to those who build tax systems that are compatible with economic growth.

Further Literature

International Federation of the Red Cross (IFRC), Welcoming a new global sustainable development agenda
www.ifrc.org/.../welcoming-a-new-global-sustainable-development

Institute for Health Metrics and Evaluation
www.healthdata.org/

Sustainable Development Goals (SDGs) - United Nations
ww.un.org/sustainabledevelopment/sustainable-development-goals

The Global Goals (SDGs), Institute for Health Metrics and Evaluation
www.healthdata.org/global-goals

Transforming our world: the 2030 Agenda for Sustainable Development
https://sustainabledevelopment.un.org/.../transformingourworld

DISCUSSION & LESSONS LEARNED

1. **Changes of donor behaviour** Location of disaster influences readiness to donor money. There is for example a great donor interest in migration around the Mediterranean region, but a small one for Subsahara and Ethiopia.

2. **Engagement of industry in humanitarian help**
The humanitarian industry has been shaped by a number of key events and moments that have given rise to its current dynamics. The private sector already has a lot to be proud of in terms of its responses to humanitarian situations. It provides generous financial donations. It mobilises its customers and the wider public to contribute to humanitarian appeals. It provides much of the logistics, transport and other services needed to move food and supplies to the right place at the right time.

3. **Shifting tasks of WHO**
WHO fulfills it´s objectives through it´s core functions:
   - "providing leadership on matters critical to health and engaging in partnerships where joint action is needed
   - shaping the research agenda and stimulating the generation, translation and dissemination of valuable knowledge
   - articulating ethical and evidence-setting norms and standards and promoting and monitoring their implementation
   - based policy options
   - providing technical support, catalysing change, and building sustainable institutional capacity; and
   - monitoring the health situation and assessing health trends." (http://www.who.int, 2018)

   The tasks must be responsive to the needs of a country or region. In the situation of crisis not only technical advices, but also "management" and coordination of other actors is required. For example the overwhelming demands of Ebola created by the outbreaks and clearly stated that WHO, acting alone, could not meet all response needs for a disease of this scale and complexity. More partnership is necessary. What is needed is an operational strategy that enables WHO to enter into public–private partnerships while safeguarding its values and improving the accountability and transparency of its operations.

4. **Changing role of the United Nations**
The United Nations (UN) since its inception has been actively involved in protecting and promoting good health worldwide. The World Health Organization (WHO) is the body of the UN responsible for directing and coordinating health. The definition of innovations seems not to be clear at the moment. The Industry signals that it is "open" for worldwide organizations like UN or WHO.

(Gaby Feldmann)

4.2.2 Health Policy in the G7/G20

The Future of Global Health Governance

Keynote 02

"Healthcare has developed into a key policy issue that is discussed at both national and international levels. In 2017, the G20 will for the first time include a meeting of national Health Ministers in a forum set to cover topics like health security and Antimicrobial Resistance.
The health governance issues inherent in the Sustainable Development Goals have underlined how increasing financial and political commitments are central to solving global health challenges which must be dealt with at the highest political level."

(World Health Summit, Berlin, Germany, October 15–17, 2017, Program, P. 86)

"Widening the Scope of Global Health research – Looking beyond G7 and G20"

Georg Schütte, Bundesministerium für Bildung und Forschung / Federal Ministry of Education and Research (BMBF), State Secretary, Germany

Main statements

- The Federal Government of Germany promotes education and research: Foundations for the future in a changing world.
- Research excellence is a must in a country whose prosperity is built on the innovative strength of its industry.
- The Internationalization Strategy establishes a basis for stronger international networking activities, because no country can master the global challenges on its own.
- The Federal Government will expand existing cooperation with emerging and developing countries and create new partnerships.
- The main role of the WHO is in: Setting the agenda of global health, coordination of international public health and health policy (analyses, recommendations, providing basic orientations, fight against diseases, epidemics and ensuring a healthy and long life).

- The wealthiest developed countries have an explicit responsibility to support the strategic approach of the WHO: Crisis prevention, strengthening health systems, advance of R&D.
- Efficient research for global health can be realized by coordinated global actions. Exemplary initiatives are:
  - "Global Antibiotic Research & Development Partnership", (GARDP), one of the most recent answer to the increasing problem of "Antimicrobial Memory Recovery Initiative" (AMRI)
  - "Program of WHO" for research and training in tropical diseases
  - "Coalition for epidemic preparedness innovation" (CEPI)
  - "Global AMR R&D Hub": Coordination, intensification, acceleration of worldwide R&D

Conclusion

"Every challenge must be met in its own specific way. Functioning initiatives can serve as a blueprint for other tailor solutions to new challenges. A wide range of options, coordinated actions, tailor made solutions to win the fight against prospective health hazards are needed."

Key Message

"Global health governance with the WHO at the helm, is (supported ...) by major political bodies such as G7/ G20. It is based on existing structures wherever possible. The challenge is to develop quick and effective solutions where they are needed.

It does not matter which of the stakeholders launches an initiative. It is important, that these initiatives are established to become universally binding."

"The New Role of Health in the G20 – Building resilience, Improving Sustainability, Assuming Responsibility"

Anna Babette Stier, Bundesministerium für Gesundheit / Federal Ministry of Health (BMG), European and International Health Policy, Deputy Director-General, Germany

Main Statements

- Global challenges such as climate change, sustainable energy supply, food security and migration do not stop at national borders. No country can answer these challenges by itself: "We have to act together!"
- The political situation worldwide needs new solutions; otherwise "threats for health".
- "We are under the obligation to take care of Global Health."
- "Regulation is not a self-seller."
- The European and international health policy for intensifying the work of the WHO provides financial and human resources.
- New cooperations and reliable long-term partnerships are needed.
- A big challenge is: resilience.

"Directions for Development Cooperation in Health: Financing Global Public Goods"

Dean Jamison, University of California, San Francisco, Professor Emeritus, United States of America

Main Statements

- Global leadership is necessary (example: tobacco control)

- Challenge: development
  - Increased recognition
  - "Learning from countries, across countries"
  - Challenge for the international system

- Progress in reducing mortality, reducing illness in LIC has been spectacular – results are the fruits of science and technology.

- Leadership of institutions like WHO, G7/G20 have the role of control and development of new tools, a major success of global leadership. Challenges to global leadership – two broad categories:
  - Increased recognition of "Antimicrobial Memory Recovery" (AMR), pandemic preparedness
  - Increasing centrality of non communicable diseases, in mortality profiles implies a learning from doing within countries and across countries is a global function.

- The biggest concern in development assistance today is, that most poor people live in Middle-Income-Countries (MICs).

- Governments do have the resources to deal with health problems, but they "do not use them".

- A rethinking of the role in global systems is required.

- There are three indicators for effective development assistance: leadership, provision of global public goods, and management of cross-border externalities (cross-border movement of pathogens, AMR).

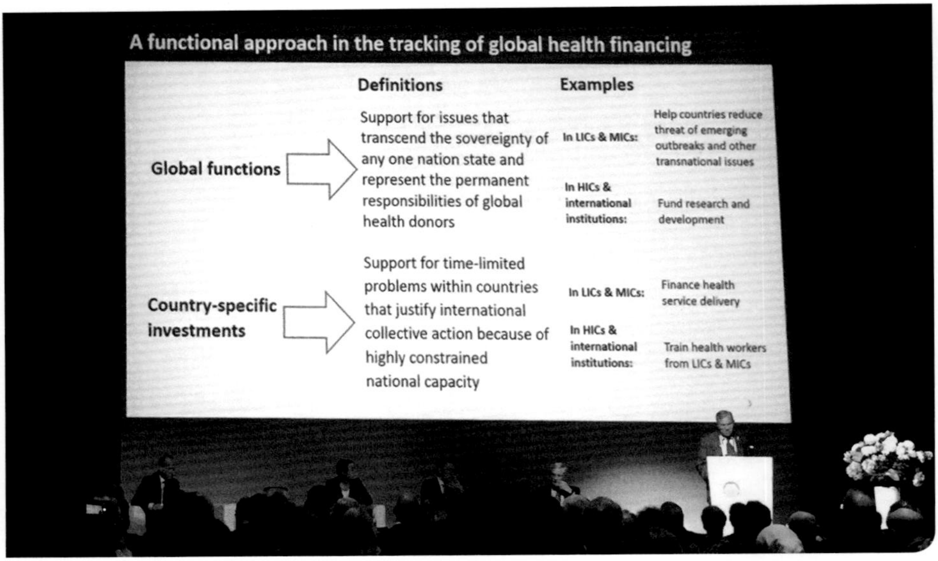

▲ *Key Note Speaker Dean Jamison presents a functional approach in the tracking of global health financing at the session with Key Note Speakers Georg Schütte, Anna Babette Stier, Neil Jordan and Chair Michael J. Klag.*

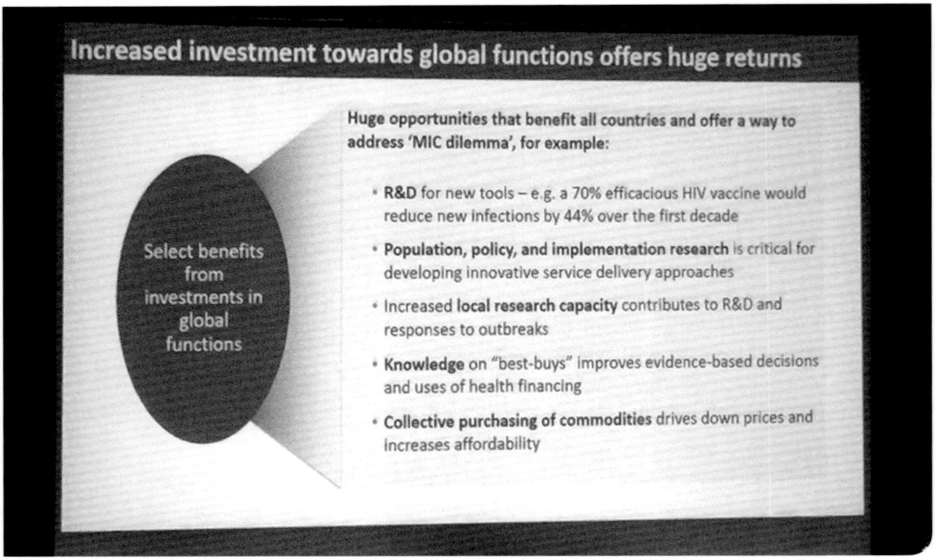

▲ *Increased investment towards global functions offers huge returns.*

Source: Health Policy in the G7/20, Keynote 02, World Health Summit 2017

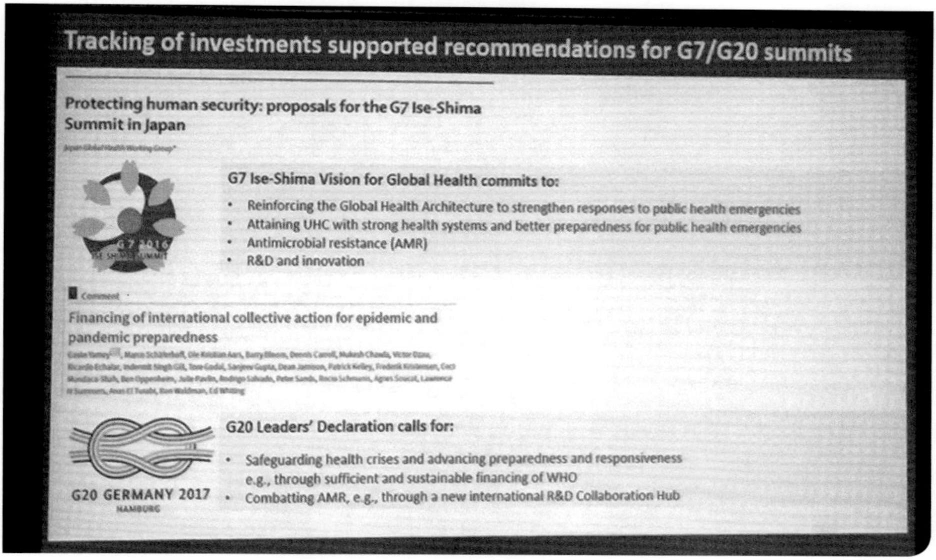

▲ *Tracking of investments supported recommendations for G7/G20 summits.*
Source: Health Policy in the G7/20, Keynote 02, World Health Summit 2017

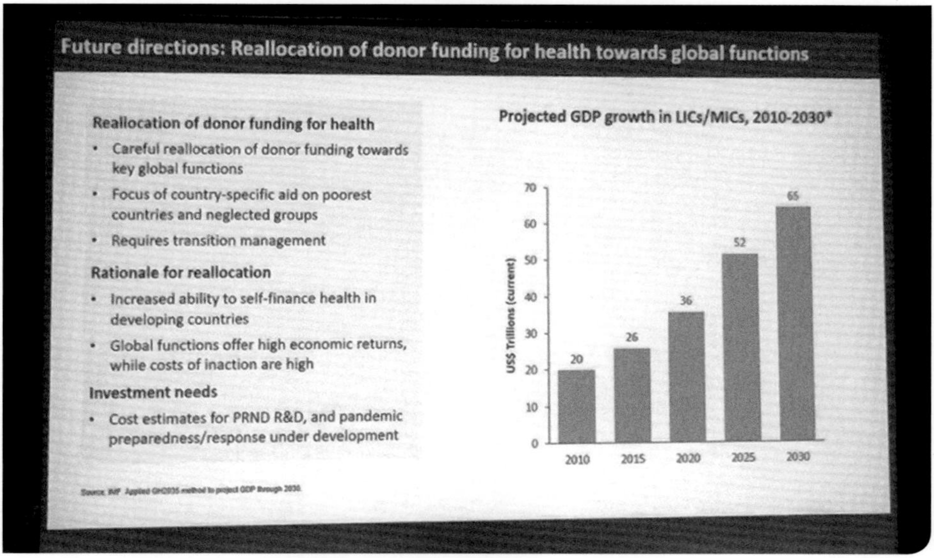

▲ *Future directions: Reallocation of donor funding for health toward global functions.*
Source: Health Policy in the G7/20, Keynote 02, World Health Summit 2017

Keynote

Neil Jordan, Microsoft, Health Worldwide, General Manager, United States of America

Main Statements

- Mission: "Empower every person and every organization on the planet to achieve more."
- Microsoft supports sustainable development goals.
- Core policies area: cloud-based technologies, new level of intelligence, commoditization, collaboration in health.
- The idea of the data donation market is based on save und trustful environment to get insights and understand the outcome of data.
- Transparent human being.

Key Message

- "We have to become more trusting and collaborative. The industry sees itself as an interface between government, academia and the industry."

DISCUSSION & LESSONS LEARNED

- Cross-border health hazards require international cooperation and international responsibility. Rather than renovation of outmoded institutional forms – which are closed, territorially fixed and hierarchical – there is a strong need to harness the power of networks, open systems and other innovations that enable new forms of collective action to achieve public goals.
- The responsibility is international, not only national.
- Human societies are rapidly evolving on a planetary scale.
- There are opportunities for global health governance to draw on institutional innovation.
- The real innovation, however, will be in mechanisms to facilitate the formation of networks, sharing of resources, generation of ideas and enabling of decision-making across constituencies that are not confined to states alone.
- The world now needs institutions that bring together expertise and ideas from far and wide, not fixed, bureaucratic and hierarchical structures which constrain how we define problems and their solutions.

(Gaby Feldmann/Delia Grün)

Further Literature

Federal Ministry of Education and Research – BMBF
https://www.bmbf.de/en/index.html

G7/G20: G7 Resources – InterAction
https://www.interaction.org/project/g7g20/g7-resources

GARDP - Antimicrobial Memory Recovery Programme
https://www.gardp.org/programmes/amrp/

Global Antibiotic Research & Development Partnership (GARDP) – DNDi
https://www.dndi.org/diseases-projects/gardp/

Microsoft Health
https://www.microsoft.com/en-us/microsoft-health

4.2.3 Global Health Financing

Workshop 17

"The objective of this session is to build an understanding about the critical importance of data transparency and accountability for global health, in particular tools for tracking global health financing, policies and strategies. The speakers come from an academic, foundation, multilateral and NGO background. They will reflect on major topics that are critical for improving global health and reaching SDG 3 ("Ensure healthy lives and promote wellbeing for all at all ages"), including global health R & D, health security, and financing for infectious diseases and reproductive, maternal, newborn, child and adolescent health.
In their contributions, they will highlight the role of new and emerging tools to increase accountability and transparency in global health. The panel will also introduce participants to the Donor Tracker, a free online resource which provides quantitative and qualitative strategic information on 14 major ODA donors. For each donor, the Donor Tracker provides data-driven insights on development funding trends, strategic priorities, and decision-making processes. It also includes 'Deep Dives' on global health, health R & D, agriculture and nutrition.
As such, the Donor Tracker is a highly relevant resource for advocates, researchers, think tanks, policy-makers, journalists and academics working in the field of global health and development. The speakers will present examples of how they have used the Donor Tracker to support their work and research."

(World Health Summit, Berlin, Germany, October 15–17, 2017, Program, P. 98)

"Introduction of the free webtool: Donor Tracker"

Chair Christina Schrade, SEEK Development, Managing Director, Germany

- The Donor Tracker seeks to advance and support progress in global development by providing advocates with easy access to high-quality quantitative and qualitative strategic information to support their work.

- The Donor Tracker is a unique online resource that offers free, independent, up-to-date analysis of 14 major OECD donors: Australia, Canada, EU, France, Germany, Italy, Japan, Netherlands, Norway, South Korea, Spain, Sweden, United Kingdom, and United States.

- Covering 90 % of the world's official development assistance

(ODA), the Donor Tracker provides data-driven insights on strategic priorities, funding trends, decision-making and key opportunities.

Key Questions of Donor Tracker

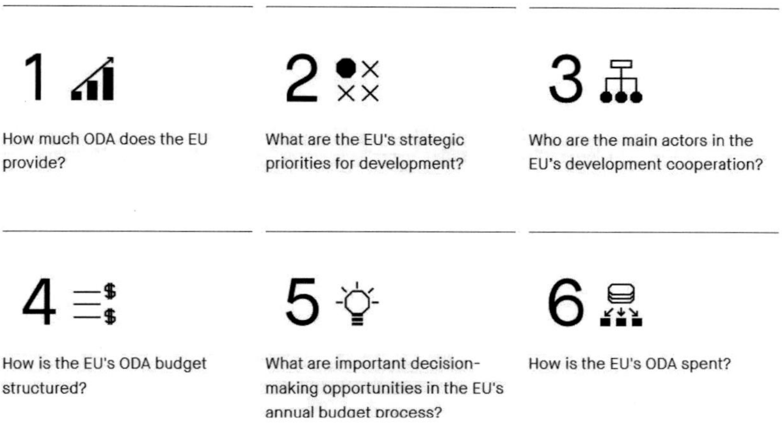
1
How much ODA does the EU provide?
2
What are the EU's strategic priorities for development?
3
Who are the main actors in the EU's development cooperation?
4
How is the EU's ODA budget structured?
5
What are important decision-making opportunities in the EU's annual budget process?
6
How is the EU's ODA spent?

Source: https://donortracker.org/country/eu

Topics of Donor Tracker

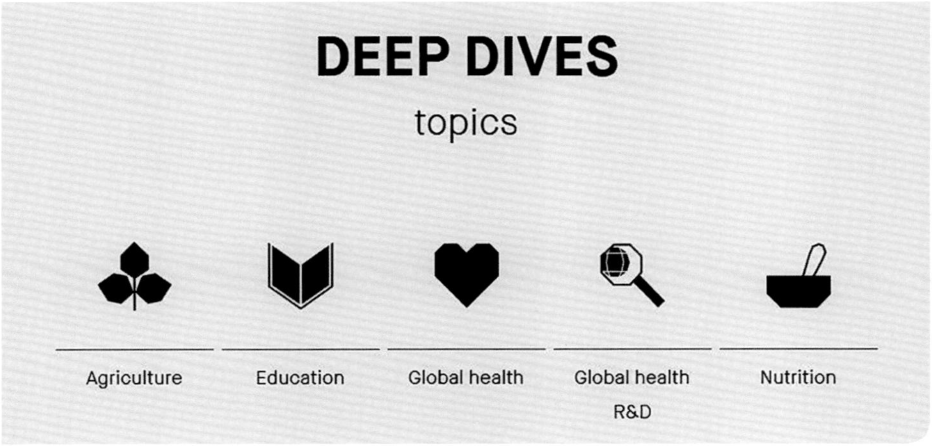
DEEP DIVES
topics
Agriculture
Education
Global health
Global health R&D
Nutrition

Source: https://donortracker.org/

"Investing in Global Health R & D"

Anja Langenbucher, Bill & Melinda Gates Foundation, Europe Office, Director, United Kingdom

Bill & Melinda Gates Foundation

- The foundation is committed to help all people lead healthy and productive lives across the globe, but mostly in regions where it's most needed to eradicate poverty.
- In Europe specifically the foundation is seeking partnerships with governments, civil society, and media to build long lasting relationships in order to improve the quality and quantity of aid spending. In developing countries, it focuses on improving people's health and giving them the chance to lift themselves out of hunger and extreme poverty.

Key Messages

- Decisions must be based on hard facts and clear data.
- Transparency is essential.
- Clear funding sources include research and diagnostics.
- Due to the fact that sources are shifting, and costs are shifting, more effectiveness is needed.

"Evidence-based and Data-driven Advocacy"

Maike Röttger, Plan International Germany,
CEO, Germany

Plan International

- Plan International is a religiously and ideologically independent aid organization committed to the opportunities and rights of children worldwide: efficient, transparent, intelligent. For 80 years, Plan has worked to help girls and boys lead a life free of poverty, violence and injustice and actively involves children in over 70 countries in shaping the future.

- Plan's ultimate goal is sustainable community development and improvement of living conditions in the partner countries. Plan responds quickly to emergencies and natural disasters that threaten the lives of children.

- Plan builds up on two main income sources:

1. Child sponsorship, to give the godchildren the chance of a self-determined childhood and a better future.

2. Single or permanent donation to one of the humanitarian donation funds or a dedicated project donation and grants from institutions and corporate donors.

Key Messages

- Plan International's accounts are independently audited.

- Exact data and transparency are required for the Donor Tracker.

- Invest in people to advocate for themselves.

"Mobilizing Resources to Finance Global Health"

Christoph Benn, The Global Fund to Fight AIDS, Tuberculosis and Malaria, Director of External Relations, Switzerland

The Global Fund Partnership

- The Global Fund is a 21st-century partnership organization designed to accelerate the end of AIDS, tuberculosis and malaria as epidemics.
- Founded in 2002, the Global Fund is a partnership between governments, civil society, the private sector and people affected by the diseases.
- The Global Fund raises and invests nearly US $ 4 billion a year to support programs run by local experts in countries and communities most in need.

Key Messages

- Donors expect high transparency. To operate with a high degree of transparency throughout the work, including applications for funding, funding decisions, grant performance, results, governance, and oversight is very important for them.
- Donors compare organizations. But it's hard for donors to understand how effective the organizations may work or compare them to other options.
- Donors want information on how the gift is going to be used. Clear information about contributions, disbursements and operating despenses must be published.

Conclusions

- Donors need data and data need donors.
- Donor Tracker is very helpful, mainly for advocacy.
- There is some scope for innovative financing.
- Data in emerging countries (e.g. China, Middle East) is not easy to get

"Promoting Accountability for RMNCAH"

Emanuele Capobianco, The Partnership for Maternal, Newborn & Child Health, Deputy Executive Director, Switzerland

The Partnership for Maternal, Newborn & Child Health

- The Partnership (PMNCH) joins the reproductive, maternal, newborn and child health (RMNCH) communities into an alliance of more than 500 members, across seven constituencies: academic, research and teaching institutions; donors and foundations; health-care professionals; multilateral agencies; non-governmental organizations; partner countries; and the private sector. Working together, the goal of the Partnership is a world in which all women, newborns, children and adolescents not only are healthy, but thrive.

Key Messages

- Align multistakeholder partner support for country-led plans across three interconnected accountability processes: monitor, review and act.
- The private sector is far from exhausted for assistance in humanitarian stressed settings.

"Advancing the Global Health R & D Pipeline"

Kei Katsuno, Global Health Innovative Technology Fund (GHIT), Investment Strategy & Development, Director, Japan

Product Development Partnerships (PDPs)

- The Global Health Innovative Technology Fund (GHIT Fund) is an international non-profit organization headquartered in Japan working with a network of partners. It invests in the discovery and development of new health technologies such as drugs, vaccines, and diagnostics. The desired returns are innovative products with the potential for game-changing health and economic impact in the developing world.

- About 20 PDPs currently are engaged in global-scale R & D (research and development) and testing of drugs, vaccines, diagnostic agents and other solutions for use against HIV, malaria, tuberculosis and NTDs.

Key Messages

- **Leveraging partners' strengths to increase efficiency**
  International cross-sector R & D partnerships in global health are on the rise. Organizations are increasingly recognizing the power and benefit of pooling unique capabilities and skills in efforts to discover, develop and deliver new health technologies more quickly and effectively. The PDP model enables significant time and cost reductions in this process through the appropriate engagement of life science companies, universities, and research institutions throughout the world at various stages in the R&D process. As a result of this coordinated network, dozens of new products have been developed by PDPs.

- **Fundraising**
  The GHIT Fund provides a platform that encourages global R&D partnerships for the private sector, enabling in companies to access global health information and assets that are unavailable domestically and reinforcing their commitment to global health in line with their business strategy in emerging markets.

Challenge: Incentive-Based Fundraising

- Modern nonprofit fundraising is more than writing an appeal letter and waiting for donations to pour in. Donors and supporters often need more incentive to support organizations. After all, their time and finances are valuable; they need to realize how the organization values its supporters and uses donations to further a cause. This is called "Incentive-Based Fundraising".
- Incentives are motivators that influence donors to give and influence fundraising teams to raise more.
- Incentives aren't just prizes or rewards; they are a means of demonstrating how much a organization values its supporters.

Recommended tool: G-FINDER

- The G-FINDER project tracks and reports on global investments into research and development (R & D) for neglected diseases. It is an uniquely informative data source, providing policy-makers, donors, researchers and industry with an understanding of the landscape for neglected disease R & D, where funding gaps exist, and how their investments fit into the global picture:
  - in 33 neglected diseases
  - across 142 product areas for these diseases including drugs, vaccines, diagnostics, microbicides and vector control products; and
  - in platform technologies (e.g. adjuvants, delivery technologies, diagnostic platforms).
  - The data includes all types of product-related R & D, including basic research, discovery and pre-clinical, clinical development, Phase IV and pharmacovigilance studies, and baseline epidemiological studies.

"Financing International Collective Action for Health"

Dean Jamison, University of California, San Francisco, Professor Emeritus, United States of America

Messages to an functional approach in the tracking financing of global health

- **There is an enormous payoff from investing in health**
  The returns on investing in health are impressive. Reductions in mortality account for about 11% of recent economic growth in low-income and middle-income countries as measured in their national income accounts. If planning ministries used full income approaches in guiding their investments, they could increase overall returns by increasing their domestic financing of high-priority health and health related investments.

- **A grand convergence in health is achievable within our lifetimes**
  We do have the financial and the ever-improving technical capacity to reduce infectious, child, and maternal mortality rates to low levels universally by 2035, to achieve a grand convergence in health. With enhanced investments to scale up health technologies and systems, these rates in most low-income and middle-income countries would fall to those presently seen in the best-performing middle-income countries.

- **Fiscal policies are a powerful and underused lever for curbing of non-communicable diseases and injuries**
  The burden of deaths from non-communicable diseases (NCDs) and injuries in low-income and middle-income countries can be reduced by 2035 through inexpensive population-based and clinical interventions. International action should focus on provision of technical assistance on fiscal policies, regional cooperation on tobacco, and funding of population, policy, and implementation research on scaling-up of interventions for NCDs and injuries.

- **Progressive universalism, a pathway to universal health coverage (UHC), is an efficient way to achieve health and financial protection**
  Two pro-poor pathways to achieving UHC within a generation can be recommended: In the first, publicly financed insurance would cover essential health-care interventions to achieve convergence and tackle NCDs and injuries. This pathway would directly benefit the poor because they are disproportionately affected by these problems. The second pathway provides a larger benefit package, funded through a range of financing mechanisms, with poor people exempted from payments.

- The international community can best support convergence by funding the development and delivery of new health technologies and curbing antibiotic resistance.
- The international community can best support countries to implement progressive universal health coverage by financing population, policy, and implementation research.

DISCUSSION & LESSONS LEARNED

- Global resources for improving health grew rapidly in low- and middle-income countries. In addition to the bilateral agencies, multilateral organizations, public-private partnerships, non-governmental organizations, and development banks that previously dominated the international aid scene, several new global health players emerged, including the Bill & Melinda Gates Foundation, the Global Fund to Fight AIDS, Tuberculosis and Malaria, The Partnership for Maternal, Newborn & Child Health, and The Global Health Innovative Technology Fund.
- More than ever, objective, comparable, and comprehensive information on national and international financial resources from all of the different funding channels is necessary to make the best decisions about where to invest and to understand the kind of impact investments are making.
- Improvements in tracking financing allow new perspectives on global health by providing key global health expenditure and payoff patterns, and illustrates the potential of the new database to inform thinking about financing reforms.
- Investment strategies are changing: public and private financing is necessary.
- Media plays an important role in creating and shaping public opinion. For low-income countries to achieve targeted health care financing reforms, the public must be well-informed on the issues.
- Corruption is a serious threat to global health outcomes, leading to financial waste and adverse health consequences.
- Donor Tracker supports evidence-based advocacy for global development. G-FINDER improves neglected disease R & D.

(Gaby Feldmann)

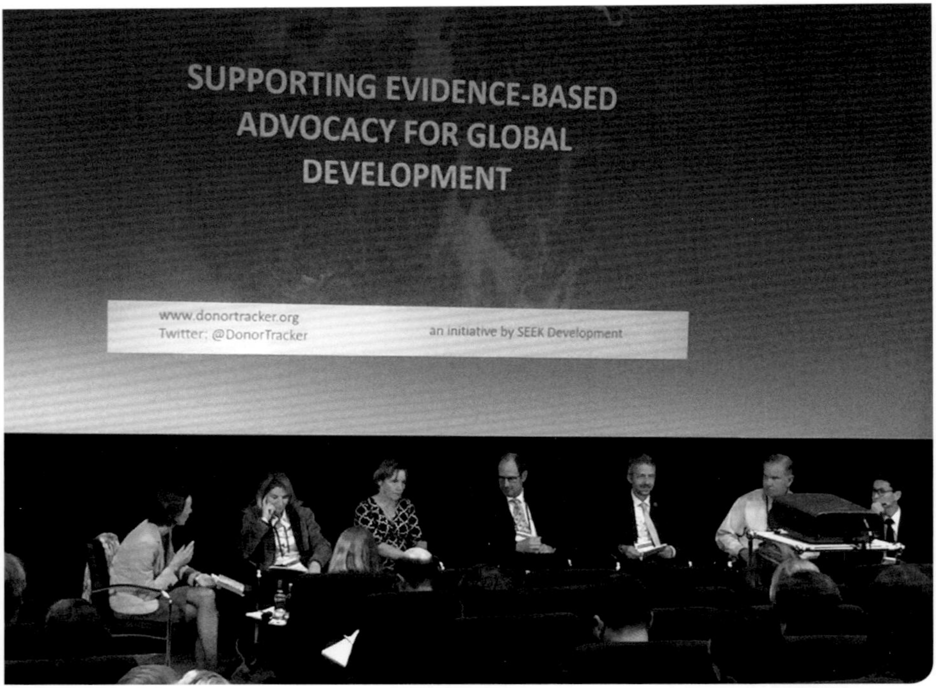

▲ *Participants of the Workshop "Global health financing": Chair Christina Schrade, Anja Langenbucher, Maike Röttger, Christoph Benn, Emanuele Capobianco, Dean Jamison and Kei Katsuno.*

Further Literature

Donor Tracker
https://donortracker.org/

Bill & Melinda Gates Foundation
https://www.gatesfoundation.org/

Reproductive, Maternal, Newborn, Child and Adolescent Health (RMNCAH)
http://www.gbchealth.org/programs/rmncah/

G-Finder
https://gfinder.policycuresresearch.org/

GHIT Fund | Global Health Innovative Technology Fund
https://www.ghitfund.org/

Financing Global Health | Institute for Health Metrics and Evaluation
http://www.healthdata.org/data-visualization/financing-global-health

Plan International
https://plan-international.org/

The Global Fund
https://www.theglobalfund.org/en/

Word Health Organization
http://www.who.int/health_financing/topics/resource-tracking/new-perspectives/en/

4.2.4 Access to Health

Supply Chain & Delivery Systems: Critical Enablers to Improving Access to Health

Panel Discussion 06b

"The global health community is increasingly focused on supply chain challenges – as multi-lateral donors disburse grant funding for commodity procurement, countries need to be prepared to efficiently absorb and utilize these funds for maximum impact. Even when procurement capacity is strong, last mile delivery challenges persist. The supply and delivery of health products and solutions are among the key challenges to access that are often overlooked. Even the most innovative and effective medicines can be rendered useless if they are not safely and effectively delivered to the patients in need.

Effectively addressing supply chain and delivery challenges requires an inclusive approach that leverages the collective expertise and experiences of diverse stakeholders. Multi-stakeholder collaborations and public-private partnerships are becoming more and more instrumental in addressing these key challenges and accelerating access to more affordable, safe and quality medicines. Equally important and often overlooked are the upstream supply chain challenges where limited collaboration among private sector companies can lead to inefficient and more expensive delivery systems.

Recognizing these bottlenecks to effective supply chain and delivery systems, 13 private sector partners came together in May 2014 to launch The Accessibility Platform. A global health initiative, spearheaded by the private sector, which aims at promoting information exchange, best practice sharing and fostering multi-stakeholder dialogue and collective actions at the global, regional, and country levels.

This multi-stakeholder panel will provide an overview of key challenges, identify potential areas for collective action and highlight best practices to jointly address supply chain and delivery issues in a holistic manner to strengthen health systems."

(World Health Summit, Berlin, Germany, October 15–17, 2017, Program, P. 128)

The panel discussion "Access to health" the panelists focused at the needs of inter-sectoral cooperation. At the end they concluded: everyone should and must have access!

The discussion started with the question: Is medicine safe?

Regulation of drugs, which reaches the market is absolutely essential. Pre-quality has to be checked as well as pricing. Currently most prices of drugs are much too high. This kind of dysregulation is shown as a market out of balance, what for more transparency is needed to get changed. A prospect for better understanding, where bottlenecks are: falsified medicine is on the market! This trouble has to be massively counteracted at once.

Too many prescriptions of antibiotics and less compliance of patients are another combat at the drugs market. These two points ends in the problem of AMR.

A question about pricing raised up in the discussion: how to inform for prices? (industry)

The design of supply chain – a simple process for the conception directly in the market was announced: how the patient is going to use the drug?

The industry of pharmaceuticals controls all steps. To get a kind of regulation, additional steps have to be included. Therefore, time is an important factor, to design the supply chain and to create different solutions (from 3 up to 20 months).

How does collaboration work? Are stakeholders beside?

Without stakeholders for example ministry of finance, it is not possible. The stakeholder's efficiency is placed in the key elements of building up own systems. But these parallel systems are a problem, because they do have a very complex own infrastructure. This is the critical aspect of collaboration: parallel systems. The claim is: one supply chain.

The private sector is not included and works on its own. To bring the different sectors together could be instructive.

The approach of sharing expert knowledge is in exit strategies in developing countries important as well. Resilient health systems need an industry with cooperation, but the way from competition to cooperation and education is a long one. A key role of the private sector is placed in training, higher education and expertise. Presented in free of charge in universities and symposiums.

Delivery systems are planned for capacity, process and orchestrate. However, a big challenge is the mistrust to the private sector. The push has to come from the countries themselves, if they need additional help.

What could be announced as success? (of course, there are different kinds of views)

- people have access to medicine
- pricing is fair
- transparency

Which steps have to be done next?

- information about disease monitoring
- implementation of standards in other countries
- no help (drugs) till now for NCDs, but e.g. malaria
- collaboration starts today, everyone plays a role
    - no one can do this on his own

In the discussion raised up the question, if a global fund for financing NCDs would be possible. Thoughts about this topic already started.

Another point of discussion was the international classification system ICD-10 and globalized use. Evaluations are currently underway to investigate the differences between regional results and impacts and misuse of the system. If there is no standard, it is not comparable. In consideration of misconduct in personal of health, no data exist as well. For improvement of public health research could be helpful.

Call for:

→ sharing the risk

→ transnational information exchange

→ trust in each other

→ transparency

Anyway, health is a driving force and the biggest economic market, but everyone has to get the possibility of access.

(Delia Grün)

4.2.5 Healthy and Resilient Cities

– Rethinking Urban Transformation

Panel Discussion 01

"Two transformative agendas come together at the city level – the new urban agenda and implementation of the sustainable development goals. Many global health actors have recognized that cities play an increasingly important role in ensuring health and well-being and responding to chronic stresses and acute shocks. A central question is how we can best achieve urban resilience, so that individuals, communities, institutions, businesses, and systems within a city are motivated to survive, adapt, and grow."

(World Health Summit, Berlin, Germany, October 15–17, 2017, Program, P. 40)

Introduction

Chair Ilona Kickbusch, The Graduate Institute of International and Development Studies, Global Health Center, Director,Switzerland

- Cities are playing an increasingly important role in ensuring health and well-being.
- The majority of world population lives in cities.
- Since 2007, the proportion of city dwellers has increased sharply compared to the rural population (mainly in Africa and Asia).
- Massive effects for human beings are chronic stress and acute shocks.
- The main question is: How can we achieve urban resilience, so that individuals, communities, institutions, businesses and systems within a city are motivated to survive, adapt and grow?

"Stress and the city"

Mazda Adli, Fliedner Klinik Berlin, Chair

Main Statements

Urbanization: "The global change in 30 years!"

Cities are good, but make us sick

- Human beings aren't well prepared to live in densely populated cities.
- Urban environment causes stress and mental ill health like schizophrenia and depression (double risk to be schizophrenic as adult of people who grow up in a city).
- To consider are a lot of social and psychological risk factors in cities.
- There is a "toxic mix of social density and social isolation" in cities.
- The key word is "urban stress". Social density causes stress, isolation, change of behaviour: irritability, higher mortality.
- Social isolation is more unhealthy than smoking or alcohol.
- Poverty around someone has an stronger determining influence than the own one. The consequence: stress associated emotional processing.
- In all of these, of course, individual differences have to be considered.

Urban advantages (e.g.)

- Cultural and social differences
- Access to development, education, welfare ...

Conclusions

- Need of "Public Health strategy for cities"
- Need of collaboration of urban planners, architects, sociologists, neuroscientists ...
- New concept "Neuro Urbanism"

"Public Health Qatar"

HE Hanan Mohamed Al Kuwari, Ministry of Public Health, Minister, Qatar

Situation in Qatar

- Diseases in Qatar similiar to European countries (overweight, diabetes ...)
- Rapid growing population (2006: 1 Mio.; 2016: 2,5 Mio. inhabitants)

Main goals of the Ministry of Public Health

- Ensuring health in the context of rapid urban development in Qatar
- Creating the platform with the result of a strong health system in Qatar

Vision and strategy of the Ministry of Public Health

National Health Strategy 2017–2022

- Leadership
- Public enagagement and support
- Health in all policies

Initiatives of the Ministry of Public Health (e.g.)

- Road safety: reducing number of car accidents, injured persons, mortality
- New campaign, new legislation concerning smoking: Shisha was not felt as a risk, "normal" (30 % of the men smoke Shisha or cigarettes)
- Network wellness center: sports, withdrawal, diet-programs
- Urban development: new healthy cities, green areas, public transport, less pollution

Conclusion

"By building new cities, we have the chance to create an environment that encourages people for a healthy life."

"The Universities Role in Addressing Urbanization and Noncommunicable Risk Factors"

Ali Jafarian, Tehran University of Medical Sciences, Chancellor, Iran

Structure of the health system in Iran

MOHME (Ministry of Health and medical education):

Executive responsibility for health and medical education (since 1985, before: Ministry of Health (1941); after the establishment of the Ministry of Welfare and Social Security, tasks related to the social security separated from the Ministry on Health in 2014

Health situation in Iran

- Strong increase in population (1900: 10 Mio., 2016: ca. 80 Mio. inhabitants)
- Strong regional differences in health
- Main problem: women overweight and obesity

Urban Health project results

- Pilot study with academic consultancy in four cities
- Education of women with major noncommunicable diseases, diabetes, cardiovascular disease, cancer etc. in residential areas (neighborhood women's capacity buildings)
- Important goal: attentiveness to become more resilient

Innovative projects in Iran

- TABASOM: women's writing project
- Iran PEN

Conclusion

"Envolving the population is the key for successful urban health projects."

"Fast-Track Cities in Ending the AIDS Epidemic"

José Zuniga, Joint United Nations Programme on HIV/AIDS (UNAIDS), Special Adviser on Fast-Track Cities, Switzerland

Fast-Track Cities Initiative

- The Fast-Track Cities Initiative was launched on World AIDS Day, July 2014, in Paris. Aim: Ending the AIDS Epidemic.

- Ending the AIDS epidemic by 2030 is feasible if the world's major cities act immediately.

Why cities?

- Rapid growth of cities
  - 64 % of population in cities in developed countries
  - 86 % of population in cities in developing countries (Asia, Africa)

- "Urban advantage": idea to mobilize cities

- The collaboration focused on 16 cities where HIV is highly prevalent.

90-90-90-Targets

Since 2014 more than 200 cities and municipalities around the world have committed to the achieving the 90-90-90 targets by 2020:

- 90 % of people living with HIV know their HIV status
- 90 % of people diagnosed are on treatment
- 90 % of people on treatment are virally suppressed
- Zero stigma and discrimination

City examples

"In Fast-Track Cities around the world we are witnessing data-driven acceleration of municipal AIDS strategies in partnership with local stakeholders, notably affected communities."

- Amsterdam (2014)
  - Amsterdam is among the first cities to have reached the 90-90-90 targets
  - wide range of HIV testing (campaigns) and health promotion
  - harm reductions services integrated into HIV strategy

- Bangkok (2014)
  - strong partnership of city society and government
  - treatment and prevention services
- Paris (2014)
- Sao Paulo (2015)

Conclusion

"Cooperation with cities concerning special diseases like AIDS or vulnerable groups shows strong positive effects."

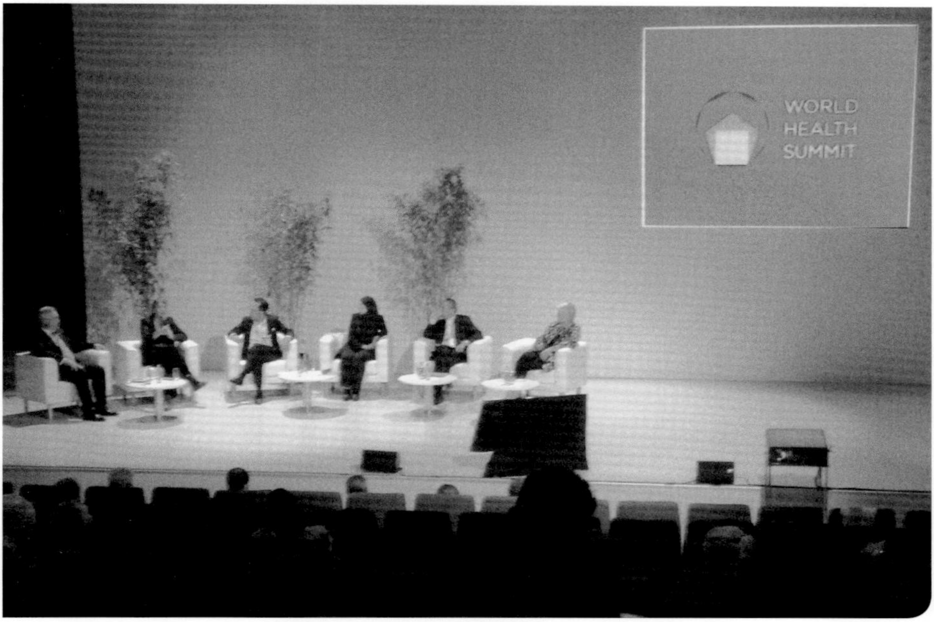

▲ *Panel discussion about "Healthy and resilient cities": Key Note Speakers José Zuniga, Charlotte Marchandise, Mazda Adli, HE Hanan Mohamed Al Kuwari, Ali Jafarian and Chair Ilona Kickbusch*

"Values of Healthy Cities"

Charlotte Marchandise, City of Rennes, Deputy Mayor for Health, and Chair of the French National Network of Healthy Cities, France

WHO Initiative "Healthy City Network"

- Cooperation of 90 French cities concerning health in the following fields:
  - Design of public areas, green areas
  - Schools (healthy lunch)
  - Streets/public transport/cycleways
  - Air pollution (public air sensors, survey stations)
  - Environment
  - Culture
  - Strong efforts for vulnerable groups

Key Messages

- Health is a political decision: "Health in all policies."
- "Empowering community leaders as health and well-being champions" is a strong asset.
- The strength of the network is crucial: "Local, national, and international stakeholders should work hand in hand."

Conclusion

Success factors:

- "Local empowerment"
- "National advocacy"
- "International connexions"

SUMMING-UP

by Chair Ilona Kickbusch

- It is banal but true, global health concerns every-day life. It also follows that there are many actors, and everyone can participate, or better, should. The government can push and set encouraging frameworks.
- Public health strategies already exist (examples from Qatar and Tehran), but "mental health must be empowered". The knowledge about these effects is still very small. This is related to stigma.
- The Qatar example shows what role health can play in politics, especially in working with local institutions. The conscious city planning can be a strong stimulator.
- Health and wellbeing are not the same. We have to clarify according to which criteria we measure them.
- The challenge and the key for health lies in the awareness of one's own health.
- Health awareness starts with identifying health risks.
- Prohibitions, however useful they might be, are out of the question in liberal societies. In order to act successful in areas of risk such as smoking and nutrition, health systems need to reach people in their worlds.
- A win-win strategy requires showing advantages, but less regulation.
- It is important to protect high risk population (e.g. AIDS).

DISCUSSION & LESSONS LEARNED

The panel discussion with experts about "Healthy and resilient cities" addresses a red-hot topic. Urbanization is one of the leading global trends of the 21st century that has a significant impact on health. Cities make up two percent of the earth's surface. Almost four billion people live in them – just over half of the world's population. Urbanization will continue. Urban populations of today and those of tomorrow are facing a fourfold threat:

- infectious diseases like HIV/AIDS, TB, pneumonia, diarrhoeal diseases
- noncommunicable diseases like asthma, heart disease, cancer and diabetes

- violence and injuries, including road traffic injuries
- and as current neuroscientific research results prove stress and mental ill health.

The factors influencing urban health include urban governance, population characteristics, the natural and built environment, social and economic development, services and health emergency management as well as food security.

Cities have to realize, that they cannot push through everything they want to.

Lobby-work is getting more important with limited advertising possibilities.

Representatives from UNAIDS, Qatar, Iran and France show promising approaches and practices of integrating health into planning, investment and policy decisions at the city level. There is a strong need for research and providing more tools.

The effect of technology is heavy: It creates benefit for the patients, delivers profit for the providers, assures equity for innovations and achieves participation of all commercial parts.

A groundbreaking example of current research initiatives is the interdisciplinary forum "Neuro Urbanism", an association of urban planners, architects, social and neuroscientists, philosophers, futurologists and odor researchers. The goal is to better understand where stress arises in the city. And how to turn cities into worth living places. There is agreement in particular in two ideas: accessible green space and places for social interaction. It is an attractive policy field and it is possible to create champions. The attention, if not the pressure of the citizens is certain.

(Gaby Feldmann)

Further Literature

Cities and politicians rally for a healthy future http://www.euro.who.int/en/health-topics/environment-and-health/urban-health/news/news/2017/10/cities-and-politicians-rally-for-a-healthy-future

Healthy city definition. WHO/Europe - Urban health - What is a healthy city? www.euro.who.int/.../health...health/...health/.../healthy...healthy

Healthy Cities https://link.springer.com/10.1007/978-1-4419-1005-9_1414

Mazda Adli: Stress and the City. Warum Städte uns krank machen. Und warum sie trotzdem gut für uns sind. C. Bertelsmann Verlag, 2017

What do you think Qatar's public health priorities should be? https://dohanews.co/what-do-you-think-qatars-public-health-prio

WHO. Types of Healthy Settings. Healthy Cities http://www.who.int/healthy_settings/types/cities/en/

4.2.6 Precision Medicine & Population Health

Forging a consensus

Panel Discussion 03

"The concept and practice of precision medicine took center-stage during the 2015 State of the Union address by U.S. President Barack Obama, when he proclaimed the goal of funding a national "precision medicine initiative." The stated mission of this initiative was clear: "to enable a new era of medicine through research, technology, and policies that empower patients, researchers, and providers to work together toward development of individualized treatments." The goal of precision medicine is therefore to approach disease treatment and prevention by taking into account the individual variability in environment, lifestyle and genes for each person.
This announcement and approach has led to a variety of responses, from enthusiastic expectation to explicit skepticism about potential health benefits, limitations, and return on investment. Will the precision medicine approach become a valuable ally in improving population health or will its effects be negligible?
The session specifically aims to see whether a consensus can be forged between these disparate perspectives on this contentious issue."

(World Health Summit, Berlin, Germany, October 15–17, 2017, Program, P. 62)

Andreas Radbruch, German Center for Research of Rheumatism (DRFZ), Scientific Director, Germany

The main aspects in applied immunology for precision in medicine are in point of view of Radbruch:

- Cells of the immune system as systemic biosensors
- Biosignatures and biomarkers for precise diagnostic classification
- Prediction of response to therapy
- Antibodies for targeted therapies
- Checkpoint inhibition (cancer)
- Checkpoint stimulation (chronic inflammation)
- Cellular therapies (stem cells, (CAR)T cells, NK cells)
- Vaccination

Tarik Möröy, Montreal Clinical Research Institute (IRCM),
President and Scientific Director, Canada

Tarik Möröy highlighted the problem, that most drugs are not effective and quite a big percentage of population is not responding to them. As well the costs which arise are tremendously. In the opinion of Möröy, precision medicine is important for prediction of responsiveness to drugs. The results of precision medicine lead to more effective treatments and reduces health system costs. As an example, he pointed out the use of a drug in case of cardiovascular disease. Afterwards the drug was taken out of market a genetic marker was detected which responded to this drug. It was shown by the specific genetic marker, that 30% of population are respondents. Möröy is calling for paying attention to genetic markers. The goals he mentioned:

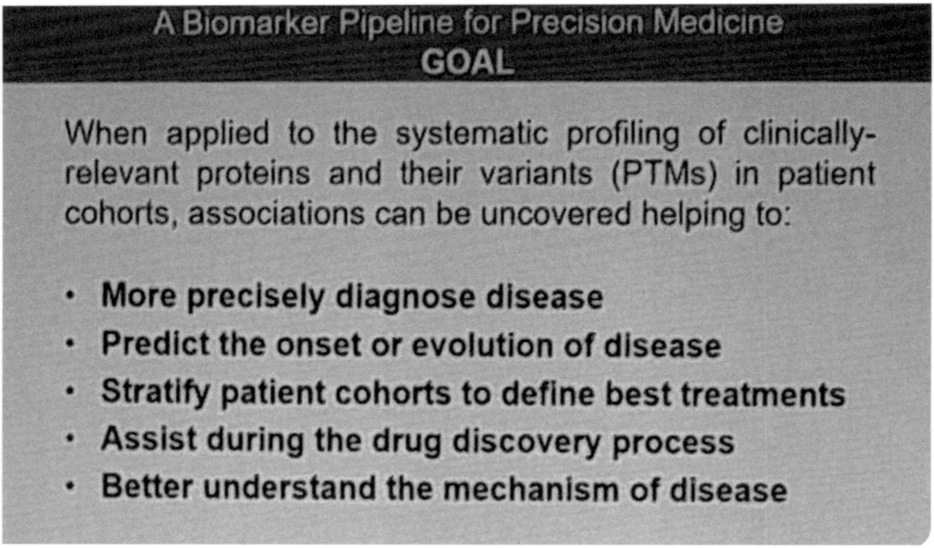

Source: Tarik Möröy, Panel Discussion "Precision Medicine and Population Health", World Health Summit 2017

Erwin Paul Böttinger, University of Potsdam, Digital-Engineering Faculty, Specialist for Digital Health, Germany

Erwin Paul Böttingers point of view is, that precision medicine and population health go together. The question of the panel to Böttinger, will the precision medicine approach become a valuable ally in improving population health or will its effects be negligible? His affirmative answer, "Digitization of healthcare will drive precision medicine approaches and improve quality and efficiency in population health management."

This can be illustrated by his presented results of APOL1, which is associated with hypertension in young african-americans (20-40y). Individuals with APOL1 expression are at high risk for high blood pressure. A recommendation can be formulated, if this marker is detected. A recommendation can be formulated, if this marker is detected. At the affected individual the parameters of high blood pressure should be screened more often. Another statement of Böttinger, genes and environment do have an impact on health. He represents the "3rd generation of health data":

- real time data, which are continuous, judicious and physiological
- Data's from: tele monitoring and sensors

Data's of the individuals are going to be directly transmitted in data health context. Currently Hasso Plattner Institute is working on realization. Their approach is the use of a data health cloud. Böttinger concludes, "together we can drive with an international partnership and community precision medicine and digital health. My argument would be, that it goes to improve population health management and enable a value-oriented learning health system."

Elena Bonfiglioli, Microsoft Corporation, Senior Director Health Industry, Europe Middle East Africa (EMEA), United States of America

A short overview of the mentioned key facts of E. Bonfiglioli:

- amount of data
- capacity and speed (things can be done)
- integration (connection of results with right solution)
- data donation

Elizabeth Blackburn, Salk Institute for Biological Studies, President, United States of America

E. Blackburn outlines two essential points:

"We must get all the data we can. From citizen to scientist, from biobanks to systems, to analyze them. On the other side – overwhelmed by data, it is very important to focus the quality of that data. High standards are needed to control."

Discussion

Precision medicine will enable to treat the patient as an individual, because of the possibility of specifying diagnostics and therapy. Therefor a big data pool is needed. That leads to the problem of the quality of data, which have to be regulated and controlled on high standards. "Garbage in garbage out", so E. Blackburn. Questions which come up to mind: How to get good or valid data? How to proof quality of data? And how to protect data? An approach of the Hasso Plattner Institute and Microsoft to face the data-problematic is the use of cloud-computing.

Another huge problem is the inefficiency of drugs. "50 % of drugs are wasted", Möröy declares. This aspect could negligible in term of using biomarkers and genetic information of the patients. A new way to discover a disease could work with catching biomarkers and genetic data. In use of looking up in clinical data, which ones are already collected and which phenotype it is associated with. The advances in electronic health data combined with genetic data and biomarkers will create progress in rare diseases, oncology and common diseases.

But how to get good data? In opinion of E. Blackburn, diseases have to be redefined, based on caught data's. The last point the panel discussion focused at, why clinical trials are not the future of treatment? At the moment everyone is treated in the same way. But individuals are responding different according to their genetic make-up. In the future it should be thought about a revisiting of the clinical trials with genetic information, which leads to new clinical trials according to genetic markers.

(Tarek)

Final statements

- Patients should be seen more as partners
- Large number of data is absolutely critical
- Health is international
- Evolution does not care about the individual, but precision medicine does

Conclusion

"We all need a little nudge."

(Delia Grün)

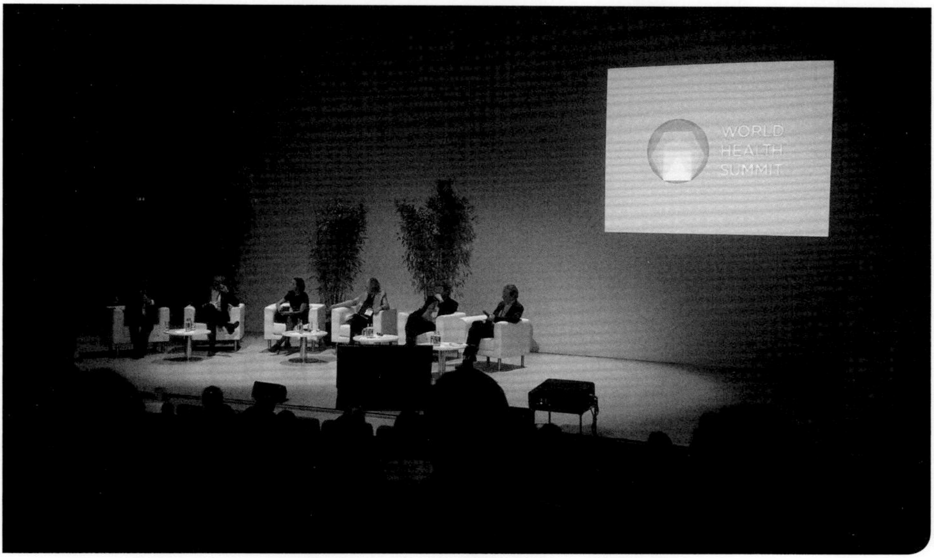

▲ *Panel Discussion "Precision Medicine and Population Health", World Health Summit 2017*

4.2.7 Sepsis and Infections in 21st century

Workshop 19

"At the beginning of the 21st century, the book on infectious diseases is far from being closed. Increasing antibiotic resistance, emergence of new pathogens, together with changes in pathogen distribution due to altered climate and mobility and the rise in the undertaking of invasive medical procedures present global challenges. This threat is further enhanced by a drastic lack of (new) effective drugs as well as by insufficient preventive and diagnostic possibilities.
In particular, vulnerability to sepsis is increasing on a global scale and is now the third leading cause of death in the world. Sepsis refers to the life threatening condition in which the body fights a severe infection that has spread into the bloodstream, often resulting in organ failure. As well as constituting a life threatening condition, sepsis is one of the most costly conditions regarding treatment, in 2011 more than 20 billion dollars spent on fighting the disease in the US alone. Inconsistency in terms of recognition and assessment of symptoms continues to constitute a serious barrier to addressing the disease.
This session focuses on the threats posed by underestimated pathogens such as human pathogenic fungi and multiresistant bacteria as well as on strategies to effectively diagnose and efficiently treat sepsis in its early stages."

(World Health Summit, Berlin, Germany, October 15–17, 2017, Program, P. 102)

At first a few aspects which have to be thought about:

- Overuse of antibiotics
- Development of new antibiotics
- Spread
- New variants

Sepsis

In general the understanding of sepsis is a poor one. Sepsis is a syndrome and it does not exist any confirmatory test as clinical argument.

Definition of Sepsis: the systemic inflammatory response syndrome that occurs during infection (Society Critical Care Medicine 2001 consensus statement).

Septic shock: vascular collapse secondary to an infectious process, usually components of hypovolemic and cardiogenic shock.

The clinical presentation depends on two main things: micro-organism (MDR, Virulence, Inoculation dose) and the host (genetic, age, comorbidity). Sepsis causes massive organ dysfunctions, that is why early recognition and intervention is absolutely necessary and lifesaving. Time is Life. The age of the patient is one of the most important points of outcome or mortality, as well as comorbidity and surgical DRG. Seasonal variations are also seen. But gender seems not to be influential.

Some aspects about the national sepsis QI-Program:

- national guideline 2014
- governmental mandated
- evidence based process
- multimodal approach to achieve process aims
  - education, leadership
  - access tool

In the national sepsis outcome report of 2016 was accounted about a 67 % increase of hospital sepsis-associated mortality trend decreases.

(https://www.hse.ie/eng/services/publications/Clinical-Strategy-and-Programmes/National-Sepsis-Report-2016.PDF)

In following refers to sepsis screening tools:

- the action sepsis 6 bundle (http://www.survivingsepsis.org/Bundles/Pages/default.aspx)
- sepsis management algorithm (http://www.survivingsepsis.org/sitecollectiondocuments/implement-pocketguide.pdf)
- maternal sepsis program (https://www.global-sepsis-alliance.org/news/2017/5/10/wsc-spotlight-maternal-and-neonatal-sepsis)

Clinical excellence Commission – Sepsis Tools (CEC)

(http://www.cec.health.nsw.gov.au/patient-safety-programs/adult-patient-safety/sepsis-kills/sepsis-tools)

→ escalation protocol// inter sectorial

→ structure of healthcare system

→ analyzing

Important for knowledge how it works, and which kinds of tests are available. But at the end there are no diagnostic tools, just pathways and guidelines for treatment of risk patients.

Other challenges in infection control is the occurrence of fungi. Fungi are pathogens for sepsis as well (Cryptococcus, Candidiasis, Aspergillose, Mucomyosis).

CDC's radar

(https://www.cdc.gov/sepsis/index.html)

- candida auris – The biggest problem, is the MDR, caused by channel strains. At the present outbreaks in hospitals are increasing. Call for: stopping the candida auris.
- Fusarium nusae – A banana pathogen, which can be transmitted to humans: human Fusariosis (Keratitis)

The problems in treating candida and aspergillus are based on increasing multi-drug-resistances (MDR), as well as azole resistance. The last named is a result of the environment, especially Agriculture and the use of pesticides. In this context the "One health" issue: humans| environment| animals, must be mentioned.

Infect control 2020:
http://www.infectcontrol.de/de/

A platform, which was initiated for research and development in identification, surveillance and combating infectious diseases.

Priority pathogens are identified and listed by the WHO, in case of COPD-Aspergilloses, AMR and TBC it already happened. Antimicrobial resistance increases since 1980s rapidly. That is one of the main causes, why the WHO calls for national action plans.
(http://www.who.int/antimicrobial-resistance/en/)

- critical priority of AMR in ESKAPE pathogens: A. baumanii, Ps. Aeruginosa, Enterobacterium (https://www.ncbi.nlm.nih.gov/pmc/articles/PMC4871955/)

- high and medium priorities

  (http://www.who.int/phi/implementation/research/WHA_BackgroundPaper-AGlobalFrameworkDevelopmentStewardship-Version2.pdf?ua=1)

Justified by the increasing multidrug resistance, new antibiotics have to be developed. Therefore, new requirements are needed:

- new mechanisms of action

- new chemical classes

- new target molecules/ pathways

Problems in Tuberculosis treatment:

Duration of tuberculosis treatment belongs 6–9 months, with a handful of antibiotics (Rif., Ison., Pyraz., Ethambutol). The main problem is focused in eastern Europe: MDR increasing!

Drugs: frontline → second line → very few new drugs are in production

But, as well in new produced drugs, first resistances came up.

An alternative is discussed in research: nanotechnology-based approach in TB treatment

(https://www.ncbi.nlm.nih.gov/pmc/articles/PMC5292193/)

Pro: better control of quality and needs

Beijing genotype: production of autotoxic stuff → cytotoxic to neutrophils → stop of production, neutrophils survival

Resolution	Goals
▶ prevention/ diagnosis/ care of sepsis	▶ sepsis six
▶ early recognition, treatment	▶ vaccination of high risk patients/ population!
▶ increase public awareness on sepsis → 80% of mortality in L/MIC	▶ Time! in treatment
	▶ global action plan on AMR

(Delia Grün)

4.2.8 Vaccination Apathy

Looking at the Non-rational Barriers to Health Protection Rational

Panel discussion 04b

"Vaccination is an effective preventative healthcare measure to help protect against infectious disease, and yet for many diseases and geographical areas, vaccination coverage rates are low. Despite the historic success of immunization in reducing the burden of illness and death, episodes of public concerns and rumours around vaccines have occurred around the world, spreading quickly and sometimes seriously eroding public confidence in immunization – ultimately leading to vaccine refusals and disease outbreaks.

This panel discussion explores the state of vaccine confidence and adult vaccination apathy, and its causes and influences. The impact of vaccination apathy is considered within the context of the globally ageing population, in light of the opportunity vaccination presents for healthy ageing.

Vaccine confidence does not solely apply to those for whom vaccination is appropriate – research has shown that healthcare professionals too are affected by negative publicity around vaccination. , With this in mind, the psychological drivers for, and barriers to adult vaccination for both healthcare professionals and the general public are assessed through the discipline of behavioural economics. Consideration is given to how a range of stakeholders, including policy makers and the healthcare community, can take learnings form behavioural science to understand and address the emotional barriers to adult vaccination, to help address the challenge of keeping our ageing population well in later life."

(World Health Summit, Berlin, Germany, October 15–17, 2017, Program, P. 94)

"The Impact of Infectious Disease in Later Life – The Need for a Lifelong Approach to Vaccination"

Horst von Bernuth, Charité – Universitätsmedizin, Head of Pediatric Immunology and Infectious Diseases, Germany

An overview about the history of vaccination of small pocks: 400,000 deaths by small pocks were counted in 18th century. The French compulsory of the vaccination of small pocks in occupied Bavaria was announced by Napoleon I. The compulsory vaccination did not exist in France, because they were not sure about the impact of this kind of vaccination. The results of the vaccination were a great success and the small pocks infection decreased impressively. In 1874 the compulsory of small pocks vaccination was done in the whole "Deutsche Reich". In 1967 a campaign of eradication of small pocks was started. In 1977 the last case was documented. 1980 the World Health Organization (WHO) could announce the eradication of small pocks.

A question which comes into mind -, if vaccination can create such great successes of eradication deadly diseases, why do we have these troubles of reliance in our societies? For example, in comparison of the expenditures of measles vaccination and the benefits of its results, the costs are negligible. Ten to fifteen persons are dying per hour, caused by a measles infection although a vaccine against measles is available. Latest huge outbreaks: California (Disneyland), Berlin (2015)

Next question v. Bernuth faced, why do we have this situation? 3,000 individuals were asked about their attitude of vaccination and why their child is not vaccinated. The outcomes of answers showed:

- 2/3 of them forgot to make an appointment or were too busy. Based on this, vaccination seems to be a victim of its success. Measles, polio and other diseases are no longer on the screen, as a threat.

- 1/3 are not completely convinced by the vaccines. This third could be convinced by arguments.

- 1 % is entirely convinced, that vaccination is amiss.

In conclusion, two-thirds of respondents could be challenged with simple recall systems and possible arguments for convenience could be:
... Non-living vaccines do not harm anyone.
... Living vaccines may harm in very rare cases.
... Wild type virus harms much more.
... The one who gets vaccinated protects others as well. For example, individuals who cannot get vaccinated, like patients on immune suppressive medication or chemotherapy.
Finally, v. Bernuth hypothesis is: Lifelong compulsory recall and information instead of compulsory vaccination will overcome vaccination apathy.

"Why do people avoid vaccines? A perspective from behavioral economics"

Douglas E. Hough, John Hopkins Bloomberg School of Public Health, Associate Scientist & Associate Director, Master of Health Administration Program, Health Policy and Management, United States of America

"At the moment there is no approach that works.", D. E. Hough determines. In the following some useful concepts in behavioral economics:

Concept	Behavioral aspect
Loss Aversion	People hate to lose
Framing	As a result
Cognitive biases	Psychology, it can lead us in particular ways – present bias
System one thinking vs. system two thinking = concept of fast and slow	Quick decision – it just felt right vs. Slow decision – it needs time and energy to change

Tools for Decision-Making in Health Care:

1. Education/ Persuasion (public health)
2. Penalties/ Rewards
3. Defaults (workplaces, schools etc. -> coming to the office)
4. Mandates (hard: "you must have to..." // soft: no enforcement // social norm – most get vaccinated)

Douglas E. Hugh concludes, success is made by how we frame it.

"Vaccination Apathy: The Role of the Healthcare Provider"

Pauline Paterson, London School of Hygiene & Tropical Medicine (LSHTM), Co-Director, The Vaccine Confidence Project, United Kingdom

Vaccination is a behavior, influenced by:

Confidence: Level of trust in vaccine or provider

Complacency: Lack of perceived need/ value for vaccine

Convenience: Access to the vaccine

A central question, what drives low vaccine confidence?

Safety concerns due to firstly coincidental rather than causal adverse events and secondly uncertainty about real vaccine risks. Less risk tolerance for vaccines than medicine is caused by visibility of disease threats and healthy individuals. The wide distrust is based in institutions like information, health providers, and scientific truths. Two other aspect which creates a low vaccine confidence are tensions between individual rights versus wider societal rights to health and philosophical or religious beliefs.

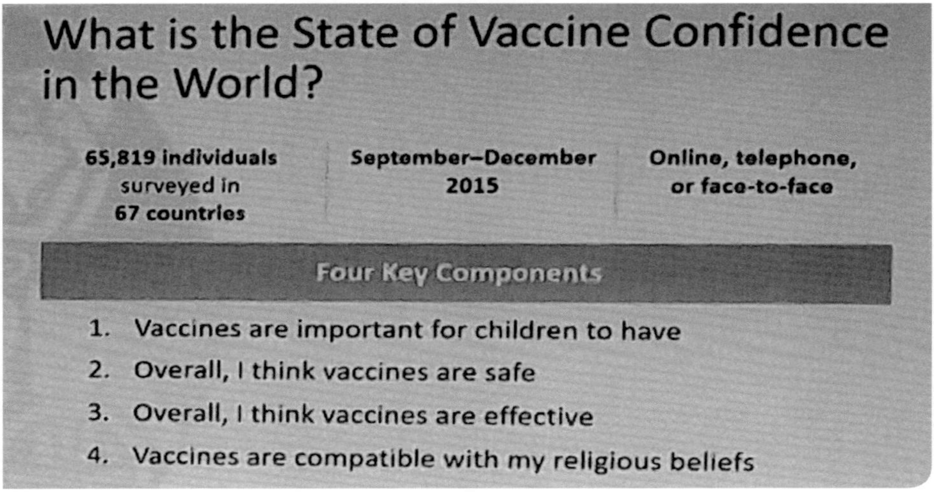

Source: Pauline Paterson, Panel Discussion "Vaccination Apathy", World Health Summit 2017

In 2015 a survey was published which faced the problems of vaccines based on focusing the topics of children's health, safety, effectivity and compatibility with religious believes. It was shown, that agreement and disagreement differ from the countries extremely. As a result, the Vaccine Confidence Index can be used as a tool to inform the design of immunization programs and strategies.

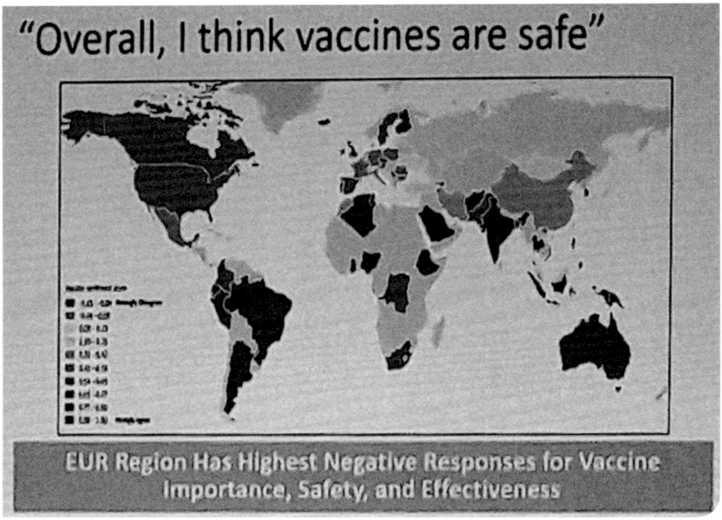

Source: Pauline Paterson, Panel Discussion "Vaccination Apathy", World Health Summit 2017

Interventions, shown to increase vaccination in healthcare providers (HPCs) include:

- free vaccine
- easy access
- educational activities, reminders or incentives
- opt outs or mandatory immunization policies
- peer vaccination

For building confidence in healthcare providers, additional training and support to aid healthcare providers in addressing vaccine hesitancy are used. As well as building or sustaining trust between HCPs, health authorities and policymakers through more shared involvement in the establishment of vaccine recommendations. Recommendation to get informed: European Centre for Disease Prevention and Control (ECDC) (https://ecdc.europa.eu/en/home)

"Three domains which have to be combated are convenience, confidence and complacency in facing vaccination apathy," Pauline Paterson emphasizes.

"Preventative Health: Vaccination as a Tool for Healthy Aging"

Jane Barratt, International Federation of Aging, Secretary General, Canada

Dr. J. Barretts points out the significant demographic transition which happens worldwide. The problems which have to be faced off are speeding up of urbanization and migration. In 2015 more than two million Syrian refugees flee to Europe. The challenges which could affect the societies are the influence of communicable diseases and infections. Another problem which was pointed out is the use of discriminating terminology especially of elderly population (cut of ages). It has to grow a mandatory for elderly population and healthy aging.

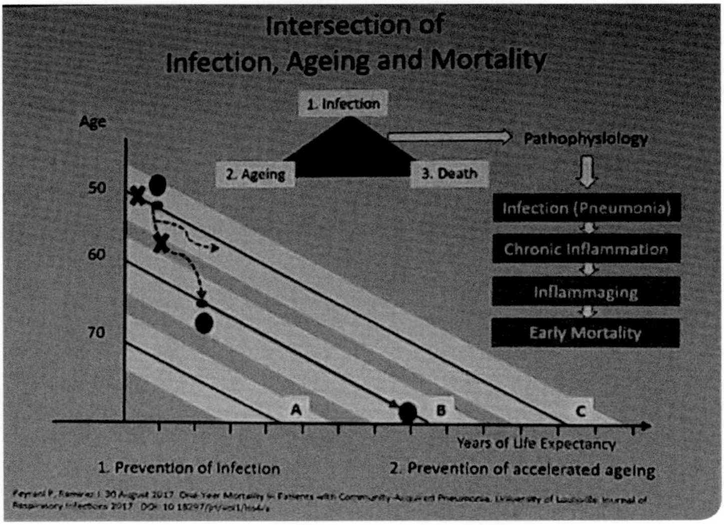

Source: Jane Barratt, Panel Discussion "Vaccination Apathy", World Health Summit 2017

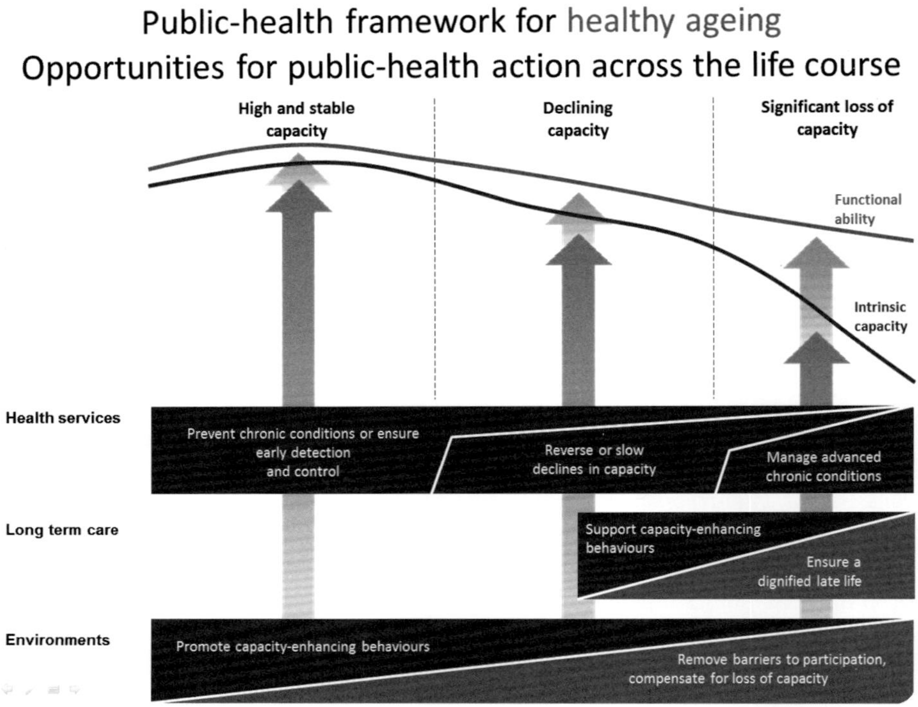

Source: Jane Barratt, Panel Discussion "Vaccination Apathy", World Health Summit 2017

Dr. Barratt calls for:

1. A life-course approach vaccination is part of a comprehensive public health strategy
2. Special attention to at-risk adult population groups
3. Challenging ageism and age discrimination is necessary
4. Multi-sectoral and multidisciplinary engagement and education is critical
5. New narrative about aging and vaccinations is essential

Another possible approach could be to implement professional healthcare coworkers in waiting rooms. Like Paterson mentioned, we need to listen to the patients about their fears in vaccination. Also, it is absolutely necessary to use a moderate language and empathy in discussions and recommendations about vaccination. Convenience and confidence are the most problematic aspects for vaccination apathy, concludes Paterson.

(Delia Grün)

4.2.9 Innovative New Ways in Fighting NTDs

Workshop 13

Neglected Tropical Diseases (NTDs) are a group of tropical infections that affect the world's poor and marginalized populations. According to the World Health Organization, more than a billion people or one-seventh of the global population suffer from one or more tropical infectious diseases.
Availability of treatment, technology transfer, scientific collaboration and knowledge sharing but also research and development are important to move forward against some of the world's most debilitating and stigmatizing diseases. Partnerships and collaborations can play a crucial role in solving intractable challenges and tackling neglected diseases. Refined diagnostic tests and techniques allow NTD-programs to achieve success. More sensibility, cost-efficiency and good partnerships among academic, philanthropic, pharmaceutical, governmental, and nongovernmental organizations are a must.
Refined diagnostic tests and techniques allow NTD-programs to achieve success. For example: diagnostic testing for lymphatic filariasis (LF) is now more sensitive and cost-efficient, thanks to a partnership among academic, philanthropic, pharmaceutical, governmental, and nongovernmental organizations. The Liverpool School of Tropical Medicine (LSTM) is working on new macrofilaricides acting through an anti-Wolbachia mechanism. Together with Abbvie DNDi is following up on screening hits for parasites causing visceral leishmaniasis and Chagas' disease, and nematodes causing river blindness and lymphatic filariasis.

(World Health Summit, Berlin, Germany, October 15–17, 2017, Program, P. 78)

"The Changing NTD Paradigm – A Core Cross Cutting Component of the SDGs"

David Molyneux, Liverpool School of Tropical Medicine (LSTM), Emeritus Professor and Senior Professorial Fellow, United Kingdom

Neglected tropical diseases (NTDs) are drivers, tracers and markers of poverty. With a "litmus" test of progress towards achievement of most SDGs. The crucial component of Universal Health Coverage is – "leave no one behind". The targets to 2030 – reduction in the number of people requiring interventions against NTDs by 90%, including effective and sustainable vector control.

Paper:
https://idpjournal.biomedcentral.com/track/pdf/10.1186/s40249-017-0288-0?site=idpjournal.biomedcentral.com

Examples of SDGs with focus on NTDS

SDG 6 Water and Sanitation In reaching the goal of SDG 6, great progress happened in case of accessibility of filters and stores for clean water. But it is still critical in focus on NTDs.

SDG 10 Reduced inequalities The "chronic pandemic" of NTDs will not disappear, if furthermore just 6% of total fund is spent in NTDs.

Paper:
http://www.thelancet.com/journals/lancet/article/PIIS0140-6736(16)30171-4/fulltext

SDG 11/13 The comeback of Aedes Aegypti, a very important vector of infections:

- Dengue
- Chikungunya
- Zika
- Yellow fever

The workshop participants and experts do agree, that new challenges are rising up, for example in case of vector control. Movements of vectors in Himalaya area from 1,000 to 2,000 meters upwards are noticed. As well the education of medical students has to be reformed. The topic of NTDs are in curriculum included, but the allowed time is far too little. The focus has to be to engage students in this topic. The inclusion of communities in innovations for planning programs, in facing NTDs already started and have to be continued. Molyneux concludes with referring to the importance of global health, climate change and vector control response.

"How to Build up New Partnerships for Innovations?"

Humphrey D. Mazigo, Catholic University of Health and Allied Sciences, Senior Lecturer, Tanzania

Human health has to be improved on various levels: local, regional and global

Mazigo points out following possible partners, who emerges:

- individual initiatives
- private companies
- research organizations and universities
- governments and donors

Phases of partnerhip building for Innovation

- Scoping
- Identify partners
- Build relationship
- Plan activities
- Create structure of partnership
- Resourcing (cash and non-cash)
- Implementing work plan
- Measuring outcome and impact
- Review the impact of partnership
- Institutionalizing = Ensuring long-term partnership
- Sustainability

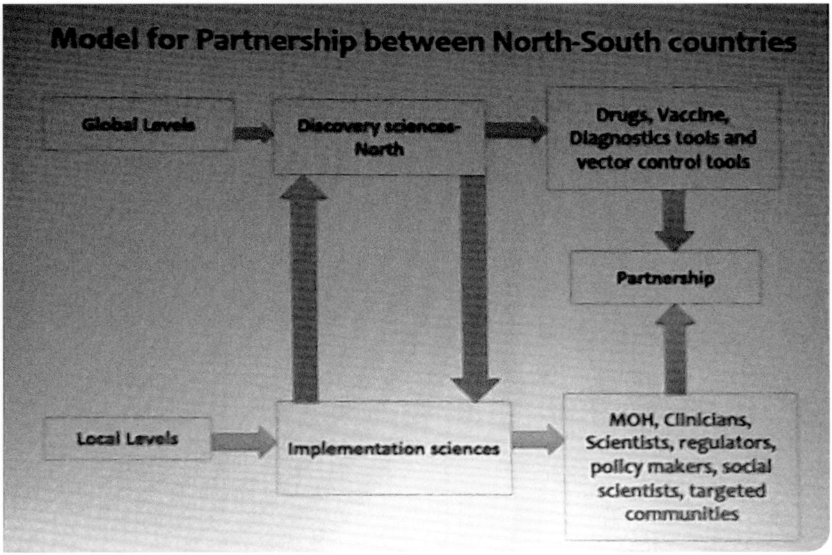

Source: H.D. Mazigo, Workshop "Innovative New Ways in Fighting NTDs", World Health Summit 2017

"What are the Challenges of the Private Sector for Fight Schistosomiasis?"

Jutta Reinhard-Rupp, Merck KGaA, Darmstadt, Merck Global Health Institute, Head, Switzerland

A company dedicated to Corporate Responsibility and Global Health

"I have always kept this passion, especially for Global Health and the African continent (...) You have my full commitment...", Dr. Stefan Oschmann Inaugural speech as CEO of Merck, April 2016

Strategic R&D framework

Intensifying control and supporting elimination agenda:

1. Merck Global Health Institute (MGHI) focuses on infectious diseases for which Merck has history: schistosomiasis, malaria
2. MGHI will expand towards other indications to address a key global threat: bacterial infections and antimicrobial resistance
3. Delivering Merck integrated health solutions, with first assets within next 3 years

Social business model ensuring sustainability, affordability and availability of products and services

1. Co-funding R&D with Global donor organizations to de-risk investments
2. PPP creation to support development
3. Partnership for implementation to ensure affordability and access

Social Business

- created and designed to address social problems
- targeting underserved populations
- ensuring sustainable and affordable access
- non-maximizing profit model

Delivering integrated health solutions addressing major global health challenges

Integrated health solutions to ensure: Impact

- Treatment: Focus on children and women

- Transmission: Development of products to improve personal preventive measures

Innovative financial mechanisms to ensure: Sustainability

- Diagnostics: Focus on highly sensitive and specific diagnostics

- Health system strengthening: Development of digital technologies and educational programs to support Healthcare systems

Conclusion

Networking is absolutely necessary for advance in research, risk sharing and reducing. It is needed to think about possibilities of win-win, by reducing the risk for the individual. Solutions could be found in building infrastructure, clinical trials and higher educational programs.

"What could be Game Changers in Filarial Elimination Programs?"

Achim Hörauf, University Hospital Bonn, Institute of Medical Microbiology, Immunology and Parasitology, Director, Germany

The goal is the elimination of Leishmaniasis filariasis (LF) by 2020. Some countries have already stopped MDA and are in surveillance phase. But other countries have not yet started. Problems which came up, evaluation units are sometimes too large and contain too many non-endemic spots. CAVE: arithmetic elimination of LF, because 60-70 million individuals are infected.

Which kind of treatment is available?
Triple therapy IDA is now being tested in large community trials (altogether > 30,000 people) for safety and efficacy. The goal is to speed up programs.

drugs: DEC/ ALB/ IVM → against larva

goal: speed up programs

Paper: https://academic.oup.com/cid/article/62/3/334/2462870

What is needed?
Drugs with adulticide activity (e.g. Ivermectin)

- new drugs

- re-purposing of registered drugs

Wolbachia endosymbionts of filarial nematodes

Symbionts are in some filarial species: O. volvulus, W. bancrofti, Brugia spp., Mansonella spp., Dirofilaria spp.

Not in: Loa loa, O. flexuosa, A. viteae, Setaria spp.

The transmission happens vertical, via oocytes and is found in hypodermic and embryos of filariae. It is associated with blindness in murine onchocerciasis (St. Andre et al., 2002)

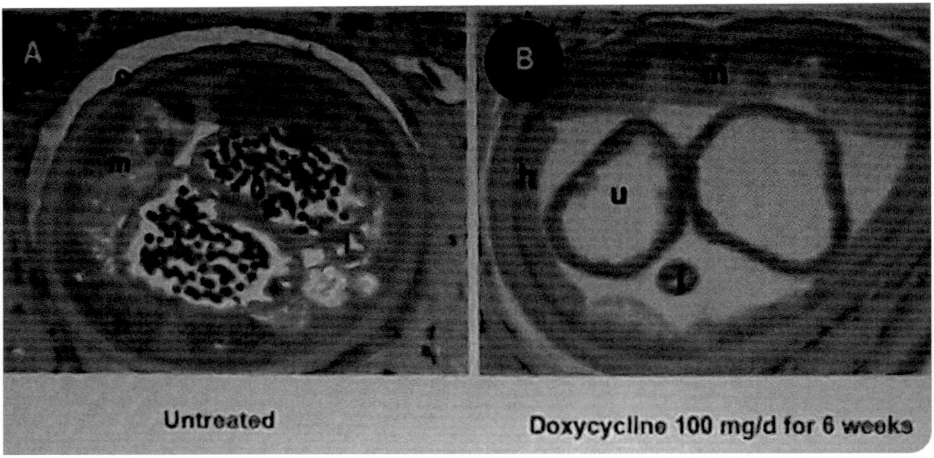

Source: A. Hörauf, Workshop "Innovative New Ways in Fighting NTDs", World Health Summit 2017

Papers: Endosymbiotic bacteria in worms as targets for a novel chemotherapy in filariasis.

(http://www.thelancet.com/journals/lancet/article/PIIS0140-6736(00)02095-X/fulltext)

Depletion of wolbachia endobacteria in Onchocerca volvulus by doxycycline and mirofilaridermia after Ivermectin treatment.

(http://www.thelancet.com/journals/lancet/article/PIIS0140-6736(00)04581-5/fulltext)

"Strengthening Capacity for Visceral Leishmaniasis Clinical Research in Africa: Challenges and Opportunities"

Monique Wasunna, Drugs for Neglected Diseases initiative (DNDi), Director, Kenya

About DNDi (Africa) – Drugs for Neglected Diseases initiative (DNDi) is a collaborative, patients' needs-driven, non-profit drug research and development (R&D) organization that is developing new treatments for neglected diseases.

Focus upon Visceral Leishmaniasis – Facts

Visceral leishmaniasis (or kala-azar), is a parasitic disease which is fatal without treatment. The disease burden is high in eastern Africa with an estimated 29,400-56,600 cases annually. In eastern Africa Visceral leishmaniasis is caused by L. donavani and affects the poorest of the poor. A 17-day combination treatment of SSG&PM is the actually recommended first line treatment by WHO in eastern Africa. Ambisome and Miltefosine are safe and effective drugs in India, but limited published data from Africa.

(https://www.dndi.org/wp-content/uploads/2009/03/Factsheet_2016_Leishmaniasis.pdf)

Call: One of the main problems is, that children are currently neglected in research.

Leishmaniasis East Africa Platform (LEAP)

LEAP – is a clinical research network that brings together experts from leishmaniasis endemic eastern African countries to facilitate clinical testing and improved access to better treatments for leishmaniasis in the region.

LEAP activities

Capacity building	Access/ Advocacy	Successes
infrastructure	community and governments	one combination treatment
trainings	media	ten conducted clinical trials
lab upgrading	LEAP meetings	over 10,000 patients treated
high standard	supporting treatment	Infrastructure development
combination treatment		800 short-term trainings
clinical research in different fields		20 long-term trainings (MSc, PhD)

Advantages of LEAP Collaboration

Combined burden of neglected diseases, can do more together with less resources. The development of regional clinical trials capacities can be used in other trials and no duplication of effort is time taken to get results minimized. The registration of much needed VL new treatments in member countries at end of study were noticed. Therefore, development of joint proposals is needed and thus sourcing of research funds is easier. Research is owned by members, hence trusted by community and governments (e.g. regulatory authorities). Governments readily give support thus translation of research results into policy easier.

Challenges of Clinical Research for Leishmaniasis – The LEAP experience	
Research capacity	Lack of/ different levels of capacity
Aligning vested interests	The collaboration brings together different cultures, environments, standards vs. self-preservation of the various institutions/ scientists
Access to treatments	Governments need to be more motivated to promote access to treatments after successful research
Tough terrain	Endemic regions are difficult to work in
Diverse research regulations	Different regulatory processes in the countries make it difficult to conduct studies

M. Wasunna sees gaps and opportunities in different areas:

- Limited critical mass of scientists in the endemic areas such as South Sudan and Eritrea. Financial resources and partnerships are needed to cover more endemic regions.
- Slow ethical and regulatory approvals as a result of divergent regulatory processes. National MoHs in Eastern Africa region to embrace regulatory harmonization strategies.
- Slow uptake of research results and translation into policy. Need to strengthen access strategies after the completion of studies.
- Lack of effective oral treatments for VL. Phase one facilities required for new chemical entities' R&D.
- Lack of appropriate treatments for patients with VL-HIV coinfection. Studies for improved VL-HIV treatments.
- Invasive diagnosis for VL patients. Partnerships with organizations such as FIND to improve diagnosis.

In the ensuing short discussion, the challenges of HIV as most important co-infection and comorbidity were pointed out. But the final conclusion is – long term partnership is useful and needed.

(Delia Grün)

Further Literature:

http://apps.who.int/iris/bitstream/10665/152781/1/9789241564861_eng.pdf

http://www.who.int/neglected_diseases/news/WHO_welcomes_new_funding_to_accelerate_demise_of_ntds/en/

4.2.10 The Health Impact of War and Terror

Coordinating Aid

Panel Discussion 06

"The role of the public health community in responding to the health impacts of war and conflict has become increasingly important in the context of the changing nature of war and conflict. While the global health community may have limited power to curb the aggression and belligerence of political and military leaders seeking out war and conflict, it can promote informed and open public debate about the causes of war and conflict by providing timely and credible information on the expected and actual health consequences of conflict. The health community also has an important role in preventing and treating injury and disease, as well as monitoring the impact and the conduct of war within the legal framework set out by the Geneva Conventions and other instruments of international law."

(World Health Summit, Berlin, Germany, October 15–17, 2017, Program, P. 110)

Christine Beerli, International Committee of the Red Cross (ICRC), Vice-President, Switzerland

The International Committee of the Red Cross (ICRC) is more than 30 years in conflicts worldwide present.

Three aspects were highlighted in focusing the impacts of war and conflicts on health:

- Interruption of supply chains
- Movement of population → care cannot be continued
- Challenge of access

Most affected fields are: regional and global health, civilian population

Currently the complexity of conflicts is dramatically increasing. Results of these processes are observed in high mortality rates of respiratory diseases, malaria and especially women are high-risk patients. As well wildfire spreads of epidemics (Jemen) and Multidrug Resistance (MDR) are rapidly growing (e.g. in Syria polio is not eradicated).

Non-communicable diseases (NCD) are huge dilemma to cope with. Most of the executed amputations are caused by not treated diabetes. Questionable are also the barriers for physicians, who are not able to reach their patients. The violence against NGOs and physicians are disturbingly increasing. In 2011-2014 were

2,400 reported cases of violence against NGOs. More and more often hospitals are becoming targets in combats. Delays in reaching the patients for ambulances are caused by checkpoints.

Call: The respect and protection of health care has to be focused and changed. Otherwise it is not possible to stop the man-made catastrophe. This work cannot be done by humanitarian helpers alone.

Axel Radlach Pries, Charité – Universitätsmedizin Berlin, Dean, Germany

The global health security is massively affected (e.g. polio is a danger):

At the moment outbreaks of cholera, measles, hepatitis is transpiring. For global health security, vector control is absolutely needed, but drugs for prevention are not available. Secondly, problems which public health in low- and middle-income countries (LMICs) have to deal with:

- maternal mortality!!
- malnutrition, caused by less production of food
- Focused on health systems, many problems are arising. At the present time reports about:
- destroyed blood banks
- main problem: HIV (central Africa)
- destroyed emergencies (Nigeria)
- no access to immune services (high risk: children)
- no training for healthcare workers

The gaps in healthcare coordination are still existing, because governments are part of these. Efforts are focused in predictable leader-, partnerships and established monitoring. It should be ensured by humanitarian aid to build up resilience.

Tewodros Melesse, International Planned Parenthood Federation (IPPF), Director General, United Kingdom

Health cluster and partnerships are part of the support of governments to health systems. To build up basic services are supported of established medical centers. The main problems they have to combat are to reach and find donors and resources.

Another point to look at is the common health is threatened. A silent killer is found in sexual reproductive health. Nonetheless, this field is not found on agendas, still now. In fragile states and conflict affected settings, the estimated lifetime risk caused by maternal mortality is 1 in 54 compared to 1 in 180 global lifetime risks.

Some reasons, why sexual reproductive health can be a silent killer:

- gender based violence (14times f>m)
- rapes
- STDs increase

International Standards

- The 1994 International Conference on Population and Development's Programme of Action
- The Sendai Framework for Disaster Risk Reduction 2015-2030
- The Sphere Project's Humanitarian Charter and Minimum Standards in Disaster Response

Minimum initial service package (MISP)

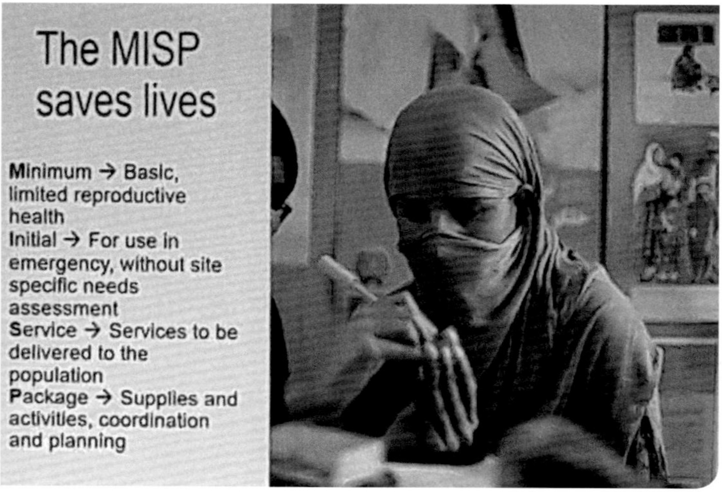

Source: T. Melesse, Panel Discussion "The Health Impact of War and Terror", World Health Summit 2017

Decrease of mortality, morbidity and disability in crisis-affected population:

1. Identify an agency to lead the implementation of the MISP

2. Prevent and manage the consequences of sexual violence

3. Reduce transmission of HIV

4. Prevent maternal and infant mortality

5. Plan for comprehensive reproductive health services integrated into primary health care

MISP is part of SPHERE and could save much more lives. Educational programs in MISP have to be extended. Around three million services were provided in MISP trainings.

(http://www.unfpa.org/resources/what-minimum-initial-service-package)

(http://iawg.net/areas-of-focus/misp/)

Syrian Crisis	Rohingyan Crisis
▶ Unwanted pregnancies and rise in STIs	▶ 519,000 arrivals since 26 August
▶ Increase in sexual harassment and exploitation	▶ "Rape and gang rape so frequent in last two years every household has a family member or neighbor who survived or someone who died as a result of rape" (CARE Rapid Gender Analysis)
▶ Early marriage has increased significantly	

Susanne Krüger, Save the Children Germany, CEO, Germany

Due to war and terror children have restricted or no access to basic needs:

- Collapse of healthcare systems
- Lack of access to food, medicines and fuel
- Attacks on medical facilities and personnel

Results are for example unimmunized children. 1 in 7 children are unimmunized and two thirds of them live in conflict-affected areas.

- 59 % in Syria
- 69 % in South Sudan
- 58 % in Somalia

Also the rising levels of malnutrition are caused by war and terror. Results are found in reduced immune systems and increased risks of pneumonia and diarrheal diseases. Malnourished children are three times more likely to die from diarrheal diseases, so S. Krüger. Also, mental health crisis will grow tremendously without treatment. The invisible wounds, will have considerable impact on children's mental health and long-term development. Last, but not least: "we cannot ignore the impact of trauma and Posttraumatic stress disorder (PTSD), if we want to build up peace. Untreated PTSD will generate an aggressive and failed generation. The global community has the responsibility to prevent this", S. Krüger concludes.

Ahmad Tarakji, Syrian American Medical Society, President, United States of America

Publications by Syrian American Medical Society (SAMS):

In "Slow Death" (2013) SAMS estimates that there are more than 640,200 people living under long-term siege in Syria, more than three times the current UN OCHA estimate of 212,00.

In "Town under Siege", Madaya July (2016), a report about 86 people, who starved to death. Three months were needed to get help of the UN.

"A new normal" February (2016), reports about increasing chemical attacks, although a resolution does exist.

Followed by a report of the current situation in Syria:

- if hospitals and health service collapse the humans are leaving the towns
- humanitarian principles do not work, because it is not the practice
- ICUs are placed in underground and caves
- small medical units go to private houses for treatment
  - health services in hospitals got too dangerous
  - hospitals are targets
  - dogs became warning systems

(Delia Grün)

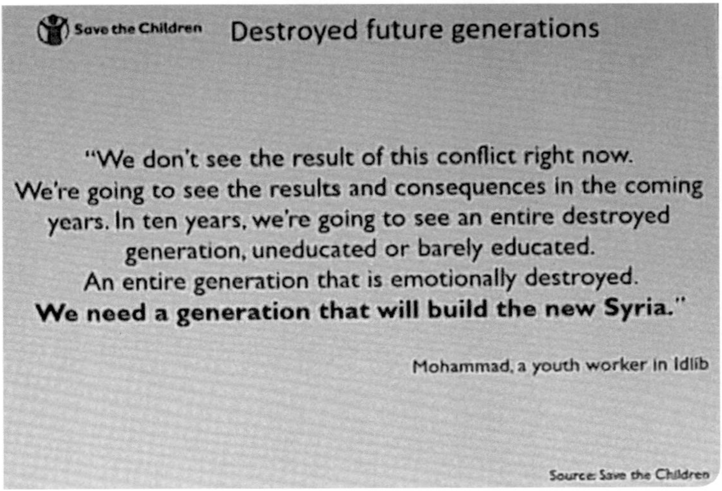

Source: S. Krüger, Panel Discussion "The Health Impact of War and Terror", World Health Summit 2017

4.2.11 Migration and Global Health Policy

Workshop 09

"The arrival of migrants from different cultures has been and continues to be a major challenge to healthcare systems in receiving countries. In particular, healthcare providers in those countries have to take into account in their daily work questions of diversity and identity in relation to their own cultural practices. This can also lead to a clash of values not least in relation to gender. Questions of perception and attitudes from both sides represent a particular challenge within the framework of globalization. This workshop aims at a taking stock of different experiments in different regions and countries having had to deal with the integration of substantial numbers of migrants. A global comparison might lead to practical conclusions for public health policies."

(World Health Summit, Berlin, Germany, October 15–17, 2017, Program, P. 64)

"The Immunization in Migration and Global Health Policy"

Giannis Baskozos, Ministry of Health, Public Health, Secretary General, Greece

Migration situation in Greece

- About 60.000 refugees stranded in Greece in 2017, most in overcrowded camps with unsanitary conditions. More than half of this year's 20.000 arrivals were women and children, United Nations data shows.
- Refugees receive little or no medical care for most health problems they face and fewer than half of those pregnant had access to maternal care. Communicable diseases, trauma related injuries and mental health problems are the most common issues facing the refugees.
- Dozens of NGOs and many volunteers provide great help for the refugee camps under adverse conditions.

Challenges of the migration health policy

- Adequate care provision
- Sustainability

Key Activity

National immunization

- Immunization is a vital component of migrant health.
- Since 2016, Greece has worked to protect the migrant population from the adversity of vaccine-preventable diseases proactively by organizing several mass vaccination campaigns. These campaigns have covered the refugee and migrant populations in reception centres. Over 30.000 doses of vaccines were provided in 2016 alone, protecting populations from ten diseases including polio, measles and pertussis.
- Those most at risk are young children who have not yet been vaccinated due to vaccination programmes in their home countries being interrupted by civil unrest and war.
- Ensuring equitable access to vaccination, including for refugee and migrant populations, is one of the key objectives of the European Vaccine Action Plan 2015 – 2020.

Results

- Prevention of epidemics
- Now explosion of mental health problems

"Migrants and Health: An Italian Perspective"

Walter Ricciardi, National Institute of Health, President, Italy

"The Italians themselves have been refugees in history. In the U.S., some of them became famous movie stars."

Migration situation in Italy

- Italy's migrant reception system is buckling under the pressure of record arrivals.
- Between 2014 and 2016, 505.000 refugees arrived.
- The problem is a European one, but it is above all an Italian one; roughly 75 % of the migrants arriving in Europe land in Italy.
- Diseases as TB, HIV and diabetes often occur.
- As recently as February 2017, migrants could access free public facilities for emergency healthcare.

Initiatives of the National Institute of Health

Two levels of action

1. **Strategy**
   It is very important to work out a transparent framework – a strategy, a scope of work and guiding principles for dealing with that recent large influx of refugees and migrants and to provide concerted support for the local governments, organizations, practitioners, scientists, professionals and volunteers.
2. **On-site measures**
   For migrants just landed on Italian coasts, health care services have top priority. It is also necessary that such services are carried out in a reasonable period of time compared to the needs identified for such a group. It is essential to carry out an initial medical assessment in order to identify cases that require specific care, more rigorous medical examinations where migrants need to be transferred to hospitals.

Results

- Guidelines published in June 2017
- Medical examinations
- Taking in charge of vaccination

"Health Care for Refugees in Berlin: Challenges and New Concepts"

Joachim Seybold, Charité - Universitätsmedizin Berlin, Deputy Medical Director, Germany

Migration situation in Berlin

- Flows of migrants and refugees at an unexpected scale not seen since the 1990s. In 2015, there were 79.000 refugees in Berlin (50 % under 15 years; 25 % from that younger than five years).

Handling of Charité

- Temporary measures to provide medical care to the refugees
- At the same time it was necessary to create regulatory mechanisms to secure the medical care of asylum seekers.
- Opening of clinics for refugees (Somatic diseases, mental health, vaccination)
- Shuttle bus from the camps for medical screening
- Medical teams (and translator) to shelter with an extra bus: examination, vaccination, reception (translation service per computer)
- Challenge mental health:
  - Culture and trauma diagnostic and therapeutic quick response in the environment with limited sources
  - Access regardless of legal and insurance status
  - Appointment within five days
  - Psychiatrics with native speaker competence and/or translator

Charite' Berlin: brief chronology

28.8.2015: Request for doctors to get involved in refugee medicine (more than 130 volunteer doctors)

10.9.2015: first refugee clinic at Schmidt-Knobelsdorf-barracks for 1.750 refugees

22.9.2015: second refugee clinic for 2 gyms (Glockenturmstraße) for 1.000 refugees

15.10.2015: third refugee clinic Registration Office

2.11.2015: fourth refugee clinic LAGeSo-premises, Turmstraße

10.2.2016: nationwide first Central Clearing Clinic to provide mental health services for refugees

1.3.2016: start of mandatory initial medical screening (according to §62 AsylG) including tuberculosis screening and vaccination

17.3.2016: catch-up vaccination program starts (shuttle bus)

7.11.2016: vaccination bus

Conclusions

- Migration is a big challenge for Public Services and Public Health.
- Significant difficulties of the Public Service and Public Health in Berlin came under the control with the support of hospitals and many volunteers.
- Systematic mandatory initial medical screening of refugees started late.
- Need for mental health care for refugees is underestimated or often neglected.

"Mobile Populations, Violence and Health"

Heidi Stöckl, London School of Hygiene & Tropical Medicine (LSHTM), Associate, United Kingdom

Human Trafficking

- Human trafficking has truly become a global threat to vulnerable men, women, and children worldwide.
- It includes a cruel spectrum of abuse and exploitation.
- The scope can only be estimated. We are dealing with a huge grey area.
- The International Labor Organization calculates that nearly 21 million people are victims of human trafficking worldwide. Roughly 55 % of all trafficking victims and 98 % of sex trafficking victims are women and girls.

Fields of Human Trafficking

- Sex works
- Domestic construction
- Manufactoring
- Industrial fishing
- Agriculture
- Food processing
- Hospitality
- Beggling

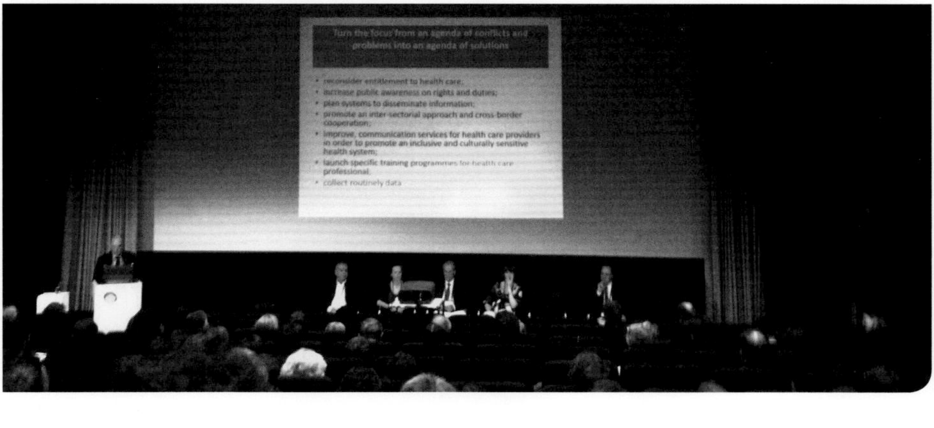

▲ *Discussion about solutions for the challenge "Migration and Global Health Policy": Joachim Seybold, Giannis Baskozos, Heidi Stöckl, Johanna Hanefeld, H.E. Reinhard Schäfers and Walter Ricciardi*

Health influences by stages of trafficking processes

- For people who are trafficked, health risks and consequences may begin before they are recruited into the trafficking process, continue throughout the period of exploitation and persist even after individuals are released.
- There is a need to highlight the migratory and exploitative nature of a multi-staged trafficking process, which includes: recruitment, travel-transit, exploitation and integration or reintegration, and for some trafficked persons, detention and re-trafficking stages.
- Trafficked persons may suffer from physical, sexual and psychological harm, occupational hazards, legal restrictions and difficulties associated with being marginalised or stigmatised.
- Policy-making, service provision and research often focus narrowly on criminal violations that occur during the period of exploitation, regularly overlooking the health implications of trafficking. Similarly, the public health sector has not yet incorporated human trafficking as a health concern.

The example Thailand

- Thailand is a human trafficking destination.
- The most vulnerable groups are women and fishermen.
- The most common violations are: Physical abuse, Sexual violence, Physical and/or sex violence.

SUMMING-UP

Chairs Johanna Hanefeld, London School of Hygiene & Tropical Medicine (LSHTM), Associate Professor of Health Policy and Systems, United Kingdom and H.E. Reinhard Schäfers, World Health Summit, Ambassador, Germany

Challenging questions

- What puts people at trafficking?
- How can people be protected?
- Which individuals carry the biggest risk?
- Which sectors have highest prevalence?

Further Literature

Charité – Universitätsmedizin Berlin https://www.hu-berlin.de/en/institutions/faculties-and-departments/charite

LSHTM: The London School of Hygiene & Tropical Medicine; https://www.lshtm.ac.uk/

Ministry of Health, Greece; https://www.moh.gov.cy/moh/moh.nsf/index_en/index_en

National Institute of Health (Istituto Superiore di Sanita – ISS), Italy; www.ianphi.org/member-countries/memberinformation/italy.html

DISCUSSION & LESSONS LEARNED

- This event part highlights the main challenges for Global Health Policy caused by the recent developments in global migration. Representatives of Greece, Italy and Germany report about their experiences in dealing with the integration of substantial numbers of migrants.

- Recently, Europe faces several societal and political challenges due to the large global migration. The current migration wave to Western Europe is a sign and symptom of the recent globalization process and the increasing political unrest. This migration is massive, unprecedented, extremely diverse and mostly unregulated.

- Arrivals of migrants from different cultures have been and continue to be a major challenge to healthcare systems in receiving countries. The health of refugees concerns everybody.

- Communicable diseases are associated primarily with poverty. In spite of the common perception of an association between migration and the importation of infectious diseases, there is no systematic association. Migrants often come from communities affected by war, conflict or economic crisis and undertake long, exhausting journeys that increase their risks for diseases that include communicable diseases, particularly measles, and food- and waterborne diseases.

- There are new challenges and emergencies within the emergency.

- Mental health problems – including depression, anxiety and post-traumatic stress disorder – are prevalent among trafficked people. There is still a grey area, based on the manifestation of the phenomenon as well the effectiveness of interventions to support the recovery of trafficked people.

- To better manage the influx of refugees and migrants an integrated solution of centralized digitalization of the data is needed.

- There are two patterns of community relationship in all countries: Manpower and NGOs.

- Parallel systems for refugees do not work.

- Migration and Health Policy remain an important task for health care systems in receiving countries and requires effective cooperation of politics and academics.

- "Migration and health are always political."

(Gaby Feldmann)

4.2.12 Big Data for Health Governance

– Benefits, Frameworks & Ethics

Panel Discussion 04

"Data is now a cornerstone of the health-care industry. It documents everything from blood pressure readings and surgical records to insurance claims, immunization histories, patient demographics and receipts of payment. But even though Big Data can bridge the gap between healthcare delivery and population health and improve many health outcomes through enhanced methods of research, the detailed collection of personal information poses ethical, regulatory and technical challenges.
This session will explore the opportunities for Big Data to assist governments and health care providers in delivering maximum benefit to society. Big Data will drive fact-based decisions by policy makers and shape how health systems address societal and global challenges in both in developed and developing economies. The increased scope, detail and availability of patient and population data will also influence the broader debate around data governance and the associated ethical issues. Our panelists will illustrate the discussion with some case studies of health data uses to help clinical practice management, surveillance, health system management, and research and innovation."

(World Health Summit, Berlin, Germany, October 15–17, 2017, Program, P. 76)

"Big Data for a Fact-Based Worldview"

Ola Rosling, Gapminder Foundation, President & Co-Founder, Sweden

Key Messages

- Dealing with data is a challenge.
- Data can be used for planning the future.
- Reliable statistics exist. There is data for almost every aspect of global development.
- "Global ignorance among the world's top decision makers in public and private sector; their global ignorance is high, just like the ignorance of journalists, activists, teachers and the general public."
- Cultural background and values influence worldview.

- It is a problem of factual knowledge. Facts do not come naturally. Drama and opinions do. Factual knowledge has to be learned.
- Education is necessary, factual knowledge has to be learned (teaching global facts in schools and in corporate training).
- "Labels" are necessary for indicating the development level of countries ("today no division of the world; most of the people live in the middle").
- People's expectations shape statistics.

Conclusion

"Data alone brings no wisdom."

"How can Big Data help to answer the Big Health Questions?"

Maxim Fedorov, Skolovo Institute of Science and Technology (Skoltech), Center for Computational and Data-Intensive Science and Engineering, Director, Russia

Big Data Definition

Big Data is data so large and complex that it cannot be effectively analysed using previously established systems, processes and resources. One of the easiest ways to understand it is by the three Vs: volume, variety and velocity.

Volume: Big Data is big. It´s analyses do not typically look at hundreds or thousands of rows of data, but rather trillions of rows, so forget desktop spreadsheets.

Variety: Big Data analyses often bring together lots of different types of data from different sources, in ways not done before. Sometimes the data are structured with clearly defined rules and logic, and other times they are unstructured.

Velocity: Big Data comes in fast and changes quickly. This type of data analysis requires processes that can incorporate newly-generated data quickly and efficiently.

This definition is extended by the two Vs value and validity, which stand for entre preneurial added value and data quality assurance.

Use of Big Data

- The collection and analysis of data of good quality are critical to improvements in the effectiveness and efficiency of health-care delivery. The so-called big data approach may allow the gap between health-care delivery and population health to be bridged and many health outcomes to be improved.

- Data-based decisions may help preventing medical errors as well identifying high risks and complement limited experience of individual professionals with comprehensive data.

- As the cost decreases of aggregating and coordinating resources and services electronically, the big data approach may deliver large benefits to low- and middle-income countries.

- The challenges of generating, analysing and applying clinical data are particularly acute in low- and middle-income countries.

- Given the sheer size of the human population and the incredible complexity of health-care delivery – with thousands of diseases and medications and interventions – the reconciliation of data-driven improvements in clinical medicine with good population health is complex.

- Sheer size increases both the potential risks and potential benefits of the approach. Although Big Data may have most value in low-resource settings, it is also most vulnerable to fragmentation and misuse in such settings.

- Collaborative governance, careful analysis and technical partnerships are needed to minimize the risks.

- In low- and middle-income countries, the shepherding of the transition from paper records to petabytes of digital storage provides another opportunity for global health institutions to offer useful governance ethics.

"Big Data in the Developed World Context"

David Delany, MD, SAP SE, Chief Medical Officer, United States of America

Key Messages

- Today data is a "cornerstone" of the healthcare-industry.
- There is a lot of data about patients in hospitals, but limited access for academics and politics.
- Providers are eager to do whatever it takes to deliver the best possible care to the patients who rely on them – but even the most accomplished and well-intentioned clinician will run into challenges if he or she doesn't have the right tools for the job.
- In order to improve outcomes end-to-end visibility across the spectrum of care at a service line level is required.
- Paying for providers to hit process gates does not secure that those gates necessarily correlate with better outcomes. We think most of them probably do, but we don't have the data to justify everything that we're asking of providers.
- As the healthcare system starts to realize the importance of using data analytics to develop this visibility into value, the marketplace will generate the tools required to innovate and make sure that every patient is receiving the best possible care along the right service lines.
- That's when Big Data will really start to line up with patient interests. Ultimately, patients want to get healthier and stay healthier in a safe and cost-effective fashion. It's the healthcare industry's job to figure out how we can do that at scale for some very complex cases across the population.
- We just need to create the guidelines and the precision around how to treat patients in a way that we can reliably follow to bring about better outcomes. That is easier said than done.
- We are at the stage of beginning to integrate this data together to get an end-to-end look across the service line. Once we have that, it's just a question of honing the data and figuring out what quality markers are really important for outcomes. Then we can take those metrics and optimize them using people, processes, and technology.

"Embedding Big Data within the Health System – Health Data Governance"

Francesca Colombo, Organization for Economic Cooperation and Development (OECD), Head of Health, France

Key Messages

- All countries can improve their health information systems and make better use of data for quality, safety and performance gains and to advance medical treatments and practices.
- Many countries are at the beginning of a complex journey to encourage the development and safe use of health data.
- Only with strong health data governance frameworks can governments safely enable data use to improve health care quality and performance.
- Eight key data governance mechanisms support strengthening national health information systems and enabling multi-country projects to improve the public's health.

Big Data provides a lot of benefits:

1. Clinical practice improvements (e.g. Israel: analytics to reduce readmissions in older patients)
2. Surveillance (e.g. USA: post-market surveillance of medical technology to improve safety)
3. System Management (e.g. THL, Finland: Public indicators to improve the quality of hospital care)
4. Research and innovation (e.g. UK Biobank: broad and deep data to prevent diagnose and treat diseases)

Risks that may arise from data uses include

1. Infringements upon individuals' rights to privacy
2. Decisions and processes that fail to respond to societal values regarding privacy and data sharing
3. Exposures of individuals to lost privacy and other harms, such as discrimination, social stratification leading to class disparities
4. Decisions and processes that weaken societal trust in health care providers and governments.

Concerns about protecting patient privacy have limited sharing of personal health data. Throughout the OECD, the legal framework for the protection of personal data recognises health data as sensitive data and therefore requires a high level of protection. To date, there is high variability across OECD countries in data availability and use.

More international collaboration is needed, in particular to:

- Support countries in developing the norms necessary for governments to certify or accredit health data processors.
- Develop guidance for the implementation of approval bodies for project requiring the use of personal health data.
- Ensure that there are sufficient agreed international standards for health data coding and interoperability.
- Support countries to evaluate which national legal frameworks for the protection of health information privacy provide adequate protections to facilitate multi-country statistical and research projects.
- Review current practices in patient consent and in waivers to consent to reach a common understanding about mechanisms that are privacy protective.
- Review developments in health data security risks and threats and mechanisms to address them.
- Explore mechanisms to engage the public in discussion about personal health data and its governance to ensure that there is good public awareness of health data, the benefits of its use, its protection, and the rights of data subjects.

"Big Data Oversight and Ethics"

Albena Kuyumdzhieva, European Commission, DG Research & Innovation, Programme Manager-Research/Ethics Review, Belgium

Key Messages

- The EU has outlined to assess an ethical dimension beyond the application of data protection rules to encourage a better informed conversation on what big data will mean for our digital rights. These are not only European issues but global concerns.

- Anonymity does not ensure privacy. This could render toothless many of the world's laws and regulations around patients privacy. Guaranteeing anonymity in exchange for being able to freely collect and use data might not be enforceable if anonymity can be hacked. Anonymization as we define it today, is inadequate and ultimately doomed to fail with large metadata.

- Public health surveillance and public health research are governed by national and international legislation and guidelines. However, many of these norms were developed in response to very different historical conditions, including technologies that have now been superseded. Such mechanisms may not be appropriate or effective in addressing the new ethical challenges

- Five key areas of concern can be identified:

(1) Privacy (including anonymisation and data protection)
(3) Ownership
(4) Objectivity
(4) Big Data Divides created between those who have or lack the necessary resources to analyse increasingly large datasets
(5) Group-level ethical harms

European Commission: Horizon 2020 Ethics Appraisal Procedure

For all activities funded by the European Union, ethics is an integral part of research from beginning to end, and ethical compliance is seen as pivotal to achieve real research excellence. There is clear need to make a thorough ethical evaluation from the conceptual stage of the proposal not only to respect the legal framework but also to enhance the quality of the research. Ethical research conduct implies the application of fundamental ethical principles and legislation to scientific research in all possible domains of research. The process to assess and address the ethical dimension of activities funded under Horizon 2020 is called the Ethics Appraisal Procedure.

= "no guidelines"

= "no whiplash effect"

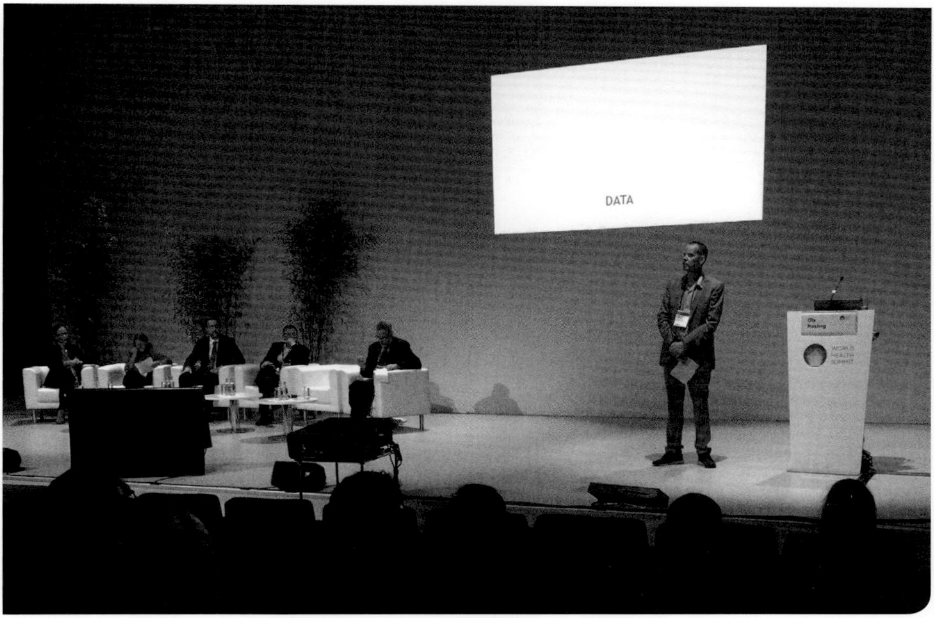

▲ *"Big Data for Health Governance – Benefits, Frameworks & Ethics" with Key Note Speakers Albena Kuyumdzhieva, Francesca Colombo, David Delany, Maxim Fedorov, Ola Rosling and Chair Ross Coppel*

DISCUSSION & LESSONS LEARNED

- Big Data is everywhere and here to stay.
- Many healthcare organizations are still struggling through this hectic phase of the big data adoption cycle, and they often feel as if they simply do not have the time, the money, or the resources for a concerted effort to make data governance a priority.
- Ignoring the role of data governance in the big data environment may be penny wise, pound foolish. Without robust, accurate, timely, clean, and complete data, healthcare organizations will not be able to move beyond the basics of record keeping and develop the analytics competencies that will become vital survival skills in the emerging world of value-based care.
- Data and information underpin nearly every activity within a healthcare organization, but some areas of operations and clinical care depend on robust data integrity and governance more than others.
- Patient safety is a top priority for every provider, and poor data governance can quickly create critical problems. From the moment a patient sets foot in the office or consult room, his or her data must be accurately identified and must follow the patient throughout every interaction.
- Detailed collection of personal information poses ethical, regulatory and technical challenges.
- Data governance is crucial for Big Data analytics, population health management, performance improvement benchmarking, and reporting for regulatory programs such as meaningful use.
- A strong governance program not only makes clinical care easier and more reliable, but will allow organizations to prepare for future analytics projects in an increasingly complex environment.
- The challenge is not just the volume. It is the integrity and the quality of that data.
- Information governance can enable trust. What will that buy? Each organization will be able to trust their data for key decision making and be confident enough to leverage that information to promote themselves.
- Big Data has the potential to transform the way healthcare providers use sophisticated technologies to gain insight from their clinical and other

data repositories and make informed decisions. To that end, the several challenges must be addressed. As Big Data analytics becomes more mainstream, issues such as guaranteeing privacy, safeguarding security, establishing standards and governance, and continually improving the tools and technologies will garner attention. Big data analytics and applications in healthcare are at a nascent stage of development, but rapid advances in platforms and tools can accelerate their maturing process.

(Gaby Feldmann)

Further Literature

European Commission – DG for Research and Innovation; https://wbc-rti.info/object/organisation/9282

Gapminder Foundation; https://www.gapminder.org/

OECD -Data-driven innovation for growth and well-being; www.oecd.org

SAP Cloud Platform Big Data Service for Health-care; https://www.sap.com/

4.2.13 Artificial Intelligence in Health

– The Beginning of a Primary Care Revolution

Workshop 06

"This session will present the views of leading change-makers in Artificial Intelligence (AI) that offer solutions for transforming health access, information and diagnostics for the wellbeing of children. The session will set out to:

1) identify avenues for achieving the vision of universal free access to quality health information and diagnostics powered by AI, and
2) demonstrate concrete examples including a short demonstration of "AI and rare diseases" through practical examples.

Questions that will be tackled:

- How can AI ensure healthy lives and promote wellbeing for all children by 2030?
- How can AI transform and revolutionize access, information and diagnostics through a multi-stakeholder approach of tech giants, startups, investors, researchers, and developers from every corner of the AI ecosystem?
- What do these solutions look like and how can they be implemented and scaled?
- What are critical issues for planning and implementing such solutions?

(World Health Summit, Berlin, Germany, October 15-17, 2017, Program, P. 56)

Introduction

Chair Stefan Germann, Fondation Botnar, CEO, Switzerland

Fondation Botnar

Fondation Botnar is a charitable foundation established with the core purpose to support children's basic needs throughout the world. It´s focus is health, nutrition and education and finances projects in these focus areas.

- Artificial Intelligence for child well-being
- Cities fit for children through smart urban planning
- Research for children
- Promoting new ideas

The foundation has supported many compelling projects over the years and is now in a process to establish a new strategy: Developing a fresh investment and organisational framework to sustainably manage the capital base.

Situation wellbeing of children

- The infant mortality worldwide is still high. In 2016, 4.2 million (75 % of all under-five deaths) occurred within the first year of life.
- The risk of a child dying before completing the first year of age was highest in the WHO African Region (52 per 1.000 live births), over six times higher than that in the WHO European Region (8 per 1.000 live births).
- The main reason is bad or no medical check-up.
- Simultaneously a global shortage of health workers occurs. Estimates assume 14 million in 2015.

Key Messages

- Innovations are necessary, both in legislation, as well as sustainability and new business models.
- The market and an enormous demand exists.
- Practical solutions for transforming health access, information and diagnostics for the wellbeing of children are necessary.

"Health Diagnostics"

Martin Hirsch, Ada Health, Founder and Chief Scientific Officer, Germany

Situation medical examination

- Usually the patient is not examined by the doctor for rare health.
- Medical examinations usually follow general patterns.
- The time for the patient is mostly short.
- Many people do not have easy access to a doctor or medical information.
- There is a shortage of doctors, especially in rural areas.

Benefits of Ada Health

- It offers a new approach to personalized health, supported by a sophisticated artificial intelligence technology (App).
- It was launched with the mission to give everyone access to high quality, personalised health information and care.
- It is a personal health companion that uses AI and machine learning to help people to understand and manage their health. Since its

launch in late 2016, over 1.5 million people have used it.

- It collaborates with the world's best research institutions to advance personalised medicine and diagnostic intelligence.

- It has been designed by a team of 100 doctors, data scientists and engineers.

- Ada's core lies a sophisticated medical reasoning engine that also supports doctors by providing earlier health information and informing clinical decision making.

- At the moment it is free of costs for the users, private financing, health insurance companies are highly interested in it.

- It is practical "democratization of medicine".

Key Messages

- Artificial Intelligence (AI) is a helpful tool.

- The future of healthcare lies in a much more patient-centric model.

PANEL DISCUSSION

Sabine Gless, Faculty of Law, Basel University, Criminal Law and Criminal Procedure, Professor, Switzerland: "Legal and Ethics in Artificial Intelligence"

Arthur Kaindl, Siemens Healthcare, Digital Health Services, General Manager, Germany: "Health Digitalization"

Hassan Mshinda, Tanzania Commission for Science and Technology (COSTECH), Director General, Tanzania: "Innovation, Digital Applications and Public-Private Partnership for Sustainable Development in Tanzania"

Martin Hirsch, Ada Health, Founder and Chief Scientific Officer, Germany

Chair Stefan Germann, Fondation Botnar, CEO, Switzerland

Points of Discussion

Artificial intelligence (AI) is not new. It was reborn three years ago and represents a transformative technology that has the potential to disrupt health, potentially more than any other healthcare technology in recent memory. In addition to the changes AI will bring in day-to-day practice, the legal, regulatory, and policy landscape will also be transformed. The following considerations were stressed:

- **Ownership**
  Data from millions of individual patients will be necessary to develop and train AI tools. Even if owner ship seems to be a concept from the analog world, it is obvious, that the patient is the owner, in clinics dispersed.

- **Safety & Liability**
  As experts cede more clinical decisions to machine-based algorithms they become inherently less responsible for the final interpretations. As a result, this is likely to mean a gradual shifting from professional liability to product liability.

- **Data security**
  The obstacles of AI in health are not solved by technology or legislation. There is no single answer but a combination of solutions: give people choice, engender public trust by appropriate regulatory and legislative frameworks, adopt appropriate technical safeguards and de-identify information at a level that minimizes re-identification risk and satisfies the specific requirements for analytics on that occasion.

- **Collaboration**
  For healthcare services to become more accessible, affordable and most importantly patient-centric, public and private partnership is essential.

- **Role of doctors in the future**
  Some fear that algorithms and artificial intelligence will take the jobs of edical professionals in the future. But instead of replacing doctors, AI can augment them and make them better at their jobs. Without the day-to-day treadmill of administrative and repetitive tasks, the medical community could again turn to its most important task with full attention: healing.

LESSONS LEARNED

- Artificial Intelligence (AI) is a red-hot topic with enormous potential.
- It is leading to advancements in healthcare treatments, such as improving the organization of treatment plans, analyzing data to provide better treatment plans, and monitoring treatments. It allows faster diagnostics reducing the time patients wait for a diagnosis from weeks to mere hours and accelerating the introduction of treatment options.
- In this day and age when people expect to get answers instantly, virtual assistants enable patients to get answers in real time.
- AI has the potential to improve outcomes by 30 – 40 % and reduce the cost of treatment by as much as 50 %.
- AI has to be reliable enough to keep sensitive data, like addresses, financial and health information secure. Institutions that handle sensitive medical information need to make sure their sharing policies keep information safe.
- Not only does AI have to be accurate and safe, it has to be created so it is up to date with new health cases. In other words, a program will only be as good as the data it learns. Programs need to be trained, or at least constantly updated, to be able to identify new/exceptional health cases.
- Since AI has not been perfected, doctors cannot fully rely on AI and still need to make decisions based on their knowledge and expertise. Patients are also at risk for the same reason. If a program provides incorrect information, patients will not be treated properly.
- The challenges for AI in Healthcare are:
  Adoption: To realize the value of AI, the healthcare industry needs to create a workforce that is knowledgeable about AI so they are comfortable using AI technologies thereby enabling the AI technologies to learn and grow smarter.

  Training doctors & patients: Learning how to use technology may be a challenge for some. Likewise, not everyone is open to information given by a robot. In other words, accepting AI technology is a challenge that needs to be addressed through education.

  Regulations: There is the need for approvals from FDA before an

AI device or application is applied to health care. This is especially true because AI is at a nascent stage and not a technology that is fully known or understood.

- Because of the ability to aggregate and analyze a massive amount of varied data, AI could yield significantly faster and more accurate diagnoses for a broader segment of the population. Individuals without access to highly specialized healthcare could gain the benefit of that experience through AI.

- Healthcare costs could potentially drop due to earlier and more accurate diagnoses.

(Gaby Feldmann)

Further Literature

Ada – Personal Health Companion App: https://ada.com/

Artificial Intelligence: How AI is transforming healthcare and solving problems in 2017: http://www.healthcareitnews.com/slideshow/how-ai-transforming-healthcare-and-solving-problems-2017

Fondation Botnar: https://www.fondationbotnar.org/en Charité – Universitätsmedizin Berlin

The Coming Primary Care Revolution: https://www.researchgate.net/publication/314111861_The_Coming_Primary_Care_Revolution

4.2.14 Innovations in Digital Health

Transforming Systems & Changing Lives

Keynote 03

"As the digital and genetics revolutions converge with healthcare into the exciting new field of Digital Health, we are increasingly able to track, manage, and improve both our own health and that of our loved ones. Digital Health is also helping to reduce inefficiencies in healthcare delivery, while at the same time streamlining access, improving quality and making medicine more personalized and precise. The essential elements that are making the digital health revolution a reality include wireless devices, hardware and software sensing technologies, the Internet, social networking, mobile and body area networks, health information systems, and genomic medicine. Like any tool, Digital Health is by itself neutral. It can either bring us closer to universal health care, or deepen the divide between the rich and the destitute, the developed and the under-developed. We need to understand how to steer Digital Health to ensure healthy lives and promote well-being at all ages and in all regions of the world. Advances are needed in issues like choosing which technologies should (and should not) be used by national health care systems in regions at di erent levels of develop- ment, on how to control complexity, and keep costs under control. Digital Health is probably the most important factor that will shape healthcare delivery in the years to come."

(World Health Summit, Berlin, Germany, October 15–17, 2017, Program, P. 92)

"From Illegible to Immeasurable – The Digitization of Healthcare"

Carla Kriwet, Royal Philips, Connected Care & Health Informatics, CEO,
United States of America

Key Messages

- Today, people are actively seeking tools and information to stay healthy and prevent disease.
- Care providers want greater insights and guidance to make the most accurate clinical diagnoses and most effective treatment decisions.
- Health systems need integrated programs to provide high quality care to more people, more efficiently.

- After a clinical intervention, patient, provider and hospital can all benefit from seamless transition to home.

Philips HealthSuite

= ecosystem of connected products, programs and services purpose-built to create smarter health solutions for consumers, patients and care professionals that uniquely spans every step of the health continuum, and every stage of a person's health.

Data from users, devices and systems is collected and compiled in an open, cloud-based HealthSuite digital platform, which continually informs the ecosystem with new insights and intelligence.

The Philips HealthSuite offers a basic structure. First connect, then more. It breathes a networked life into its new generation of devices. An obscure scale or a pure sphygmomanometer is basically old iron.

Advantages of Digital Health

- Consumers are empowered to take control of their own health and wellness.
- Providers are more connected at the point of care.
- Health systems are able to leverage informatics and analytics to deliver more personalized care across entire populations.

"EU Action on Digital Transformation of Health and Care"

Elmar Nimmesgern, European Commission, Deputy Head of Unit Innovative and Personalised Medicine, Belgium

The Digital Single Market strategy (May 2015):

- Aims to open up digital opportunities for people and business.
- Enhance Europe's position as a world leader in the digital economy.
- The Digital Single Market Strategy is built on three pillars:

1. Access: Better access for consumers and businesses to digital goods and services across Europe.
2. Environment: Creating the right conditions and a level playing field for digital networks and innovative services to flourish.
3. Economy & Society: Maximising the growth potential of the digital economy.

On May 10th 2017 the Commission published the mid-term review of the Digital Single Market Strategy. It shows the progress made in implementing the Strategy since 2015 and where further actions are needed.

The European Commission has identified the completion of the Digital Single Market (DSM) as one of its ten political priorities.

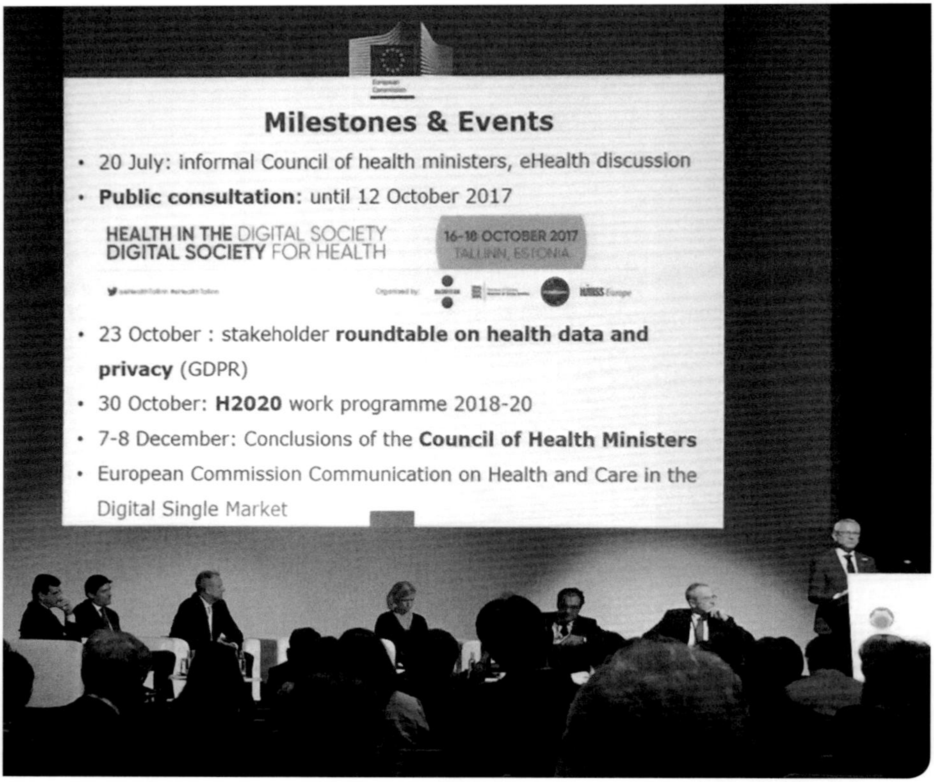

▲ *Presentation of EU Milestones & Events in "Key 03 Innovations in Digital Health": Chair Adalberto Campos Fernandes, Speakers Thomas P. Laur, Steven Hildemann, Carla Kriwet, Arnaud Bernaert, João Gabriel Silva and Elmar Nimmersgern*

"Unleashing the Power of Digital: A Technologist's View of Data-Driven Innovation in Healthcare"

Thomas P. Laur, SAP SE, President of SAP Health, United States of America

Key Messages

- Technology has had an undeniable impact on our lives and for the most part it has made our lives easier.
- We have not yet seen the full impact of digital in healthcare.
- The focus on treatment has resulted in an innovation that has been really focused on tools, devices and hardware, but not on software.
- This immaturity limits collaboration.
- Recommendations:
    - You have to break up the status quo by data-driven decisions. This starts by recognizing and respecting data as a first-class asset. Building a data governance process a consistent framework on how data will be collected, managed and shared across the organization.
    - Connect to all data irrespective of the format or the source system.
    - Democratize the data. Make it available across the organization to foster a culture of data-driven decisions.
    - Put the patient at the center.

Conclusion

True disruptive innovation from digital in healthcare will come from deeper collaboration models.

"Unlocking Tomorrow's Cures – Digitalization in the Pharmaceutical Industry"

Steven Hildemann, Merck, Global Chief Medical Officer, Head of Global Medical Affairs and Patient Safety, Germany

Key Messages

There are four main areas where digital developments will drive value for pharma companies:

- An ability to deliver more personalized patient care is a key value driver from digital technology in any industry and pharma as well.
- Engage more fully with physicians and patients.
- Use data to drive superior insight and decision making.
- Transform business processes to provide real-time responsiveness and "real world" settings.

Conclusion

Big data has already transformed almost every aspect of life, and healthcare is no exception. Data-driven healthcare is an idea whose time has come. Advances in data collection, storage and analytics have been accompanied by the proliferation of data – for example, from sensors and devices, clinical information systems and electronic health records. At the same time, data standards and interoperability are becoming more widespread, allowing developers to find more applications for health data.

Further Literature

Definition of Digital Health - Paul Sonnier - Story of Digital Health: https://storyofdigitalhealth.com/definition/

Merck - There is no innovation today without a digital component and vice versa: https://innoboard.de/.../christoph-huels-merck-innovation-digitiza..

Philips Future Health Index Reveals Perception of Health: https://www.businesswire.com/.../Philips-Future- Health-Index-Reveals-Perception

The Democratization of Healthcare Data Analytics: https://blogs.sap.com/.../the-democratization-of-healthcare-data-analytics

Transformation of Health and Care: https://ec.europa.eu/digital-single-market/en/policies/ehealth

DISCUSSION & LESSONS LEARNED

The digital future of health has only just begun!

- Although digitalization in healthcare has so far only been incremental, digital transformation has a central role to play in Global Health over the next decade.
- Data-driven healthcare has the potential to save lives and billions of dollars from health budgets but challenges relating to the collection, sharing and interoperability of medical data need to be overcome first.
- Digital health has emerged to enable approaches that are dramatically more cost-effective by reducing the frequency of inappropriate interventions.
- The investment focus will change from clinics to mobile health technology. By shifting care out of the hospital, virtual care (care anywhere) and connected home initiatives can broaden access to healthcare.
- Digital technologies have many positive aspects but also one needs to be aware of and plan to overcome the challenges related to security, privacy and integrity.
- Data Governance and Data Management are the keywords here. If data is one of the most important resources of Global Health, then formal guidance on how to handle the data is a strategic investment.
- Health care being one of the largest industries in the world is dominated by global players as market leaders.
- Transparency is a path to improve patient safety but at the same time it opens many doors for abuse. Even when records are deidentified, there remains a small risk that privacy will be compromised at some point. At a minimum, individuals must consent to surrender their information with the understanding that others may profit financially from it.
- The commercial and non-commercial use of digitized health data holds enormous potential for advances in global health, but the process will be neither straightforward nor without costs. Even you may be able to calculate the value of digital health investments by some highly-publicized measures and a probability of realizing maximum future value – for poor countries are those investments a matter of affordability.
- Access to hardware and software is still a significant problem in many regions of the world.

(Gaby Feldmann)

4.3 Startup Track

"The World Health Summit Startup Track highlights outstanding ideas and innovative business concepts, that have the potential to revolutionize healthcare and improve global health. Attending the World Health Summit provides young entrepreneurs with three days of access to world leaders in science, industry and politics to set up future collaborations and get to know potential mentors, investors and advisory board members." (https://www.worldhealthsummit.org/whs-2018/startup-track.html).

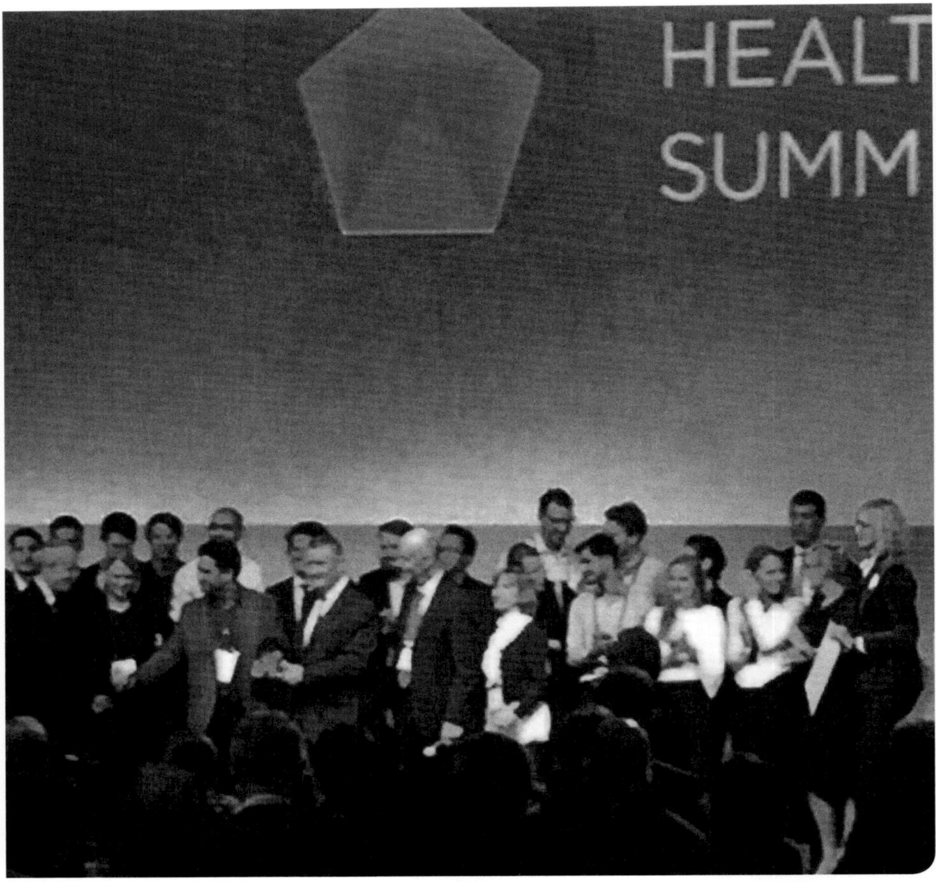

▲ *Congratulations from the German Federal Minister of Health Hermann Gröhe to Asher Hasan of doctHERs, who won the "Startup Award 2017". His idea of digitally connecting female healthworkers in rural areas convinced the jury.*

4.4 New Voices in Global Health

The New Voices in Global Health initiative promote the active participation of young scientists in the World Health Summit.

The highly qualified women and men come from all over the world and find new ways of sharing knowledge and practice.

(Gaby Feldmann)

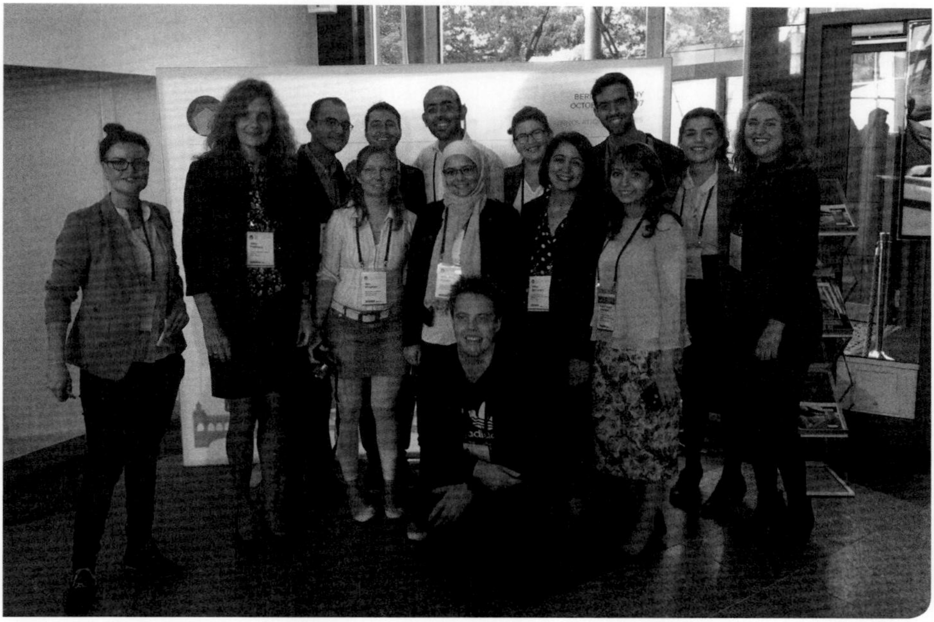

▲ *The New Voices in Global Health (NVGH) initiative present their work at the World Health Summit in Berlin (selected participants with Gaby Feldmann and Delia Grün, Akkon University for Human Sciences, Berlin)*

4.5 First year student's view on The World Health Summit 2017

Introduction

Nobel prizewinners (Elizabeth Blackburn, Roger D. Kornberg), Ministers of Health Hanan Mohamed Al-Kuwari, Qatar, Adalberto Campuos Fernandes, Portugal, and Hermann Gröhe, Germany), CEOs of well known international players (Bayer AG, Werner Baumann; Pfizer Germany, Peter Albiez), leaders of important non-governmental organizations (Joanne Liu, Doctors without Borders, Switzerland; Kevin Watkins, Save the Children, UK) and many other decision makers and representatives from policy, academia, private sector and civil society worldwide met on the occasion of the World Health Summit 2017. Between the 2.000 participants – me: a first year student of International Emergency and Disaster Management at the Akkon University for Human Sciences, Berlin – yet without any professional medical background but eager to learn.

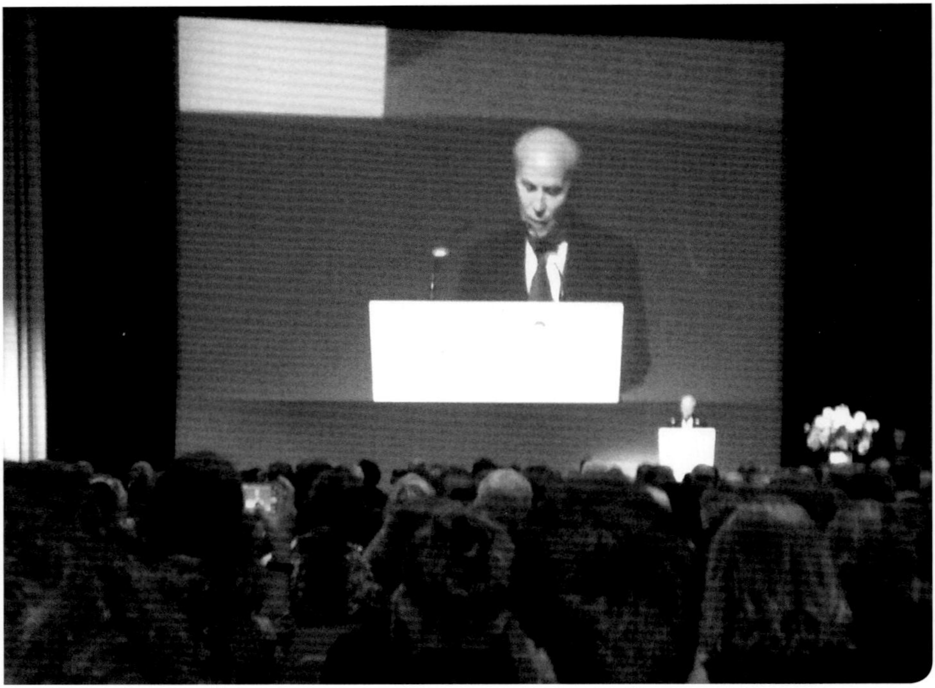

▲ *Prominent speakers at the World Health Summit 2017; here Nobel prizewinner Roger D. Kornberg.*

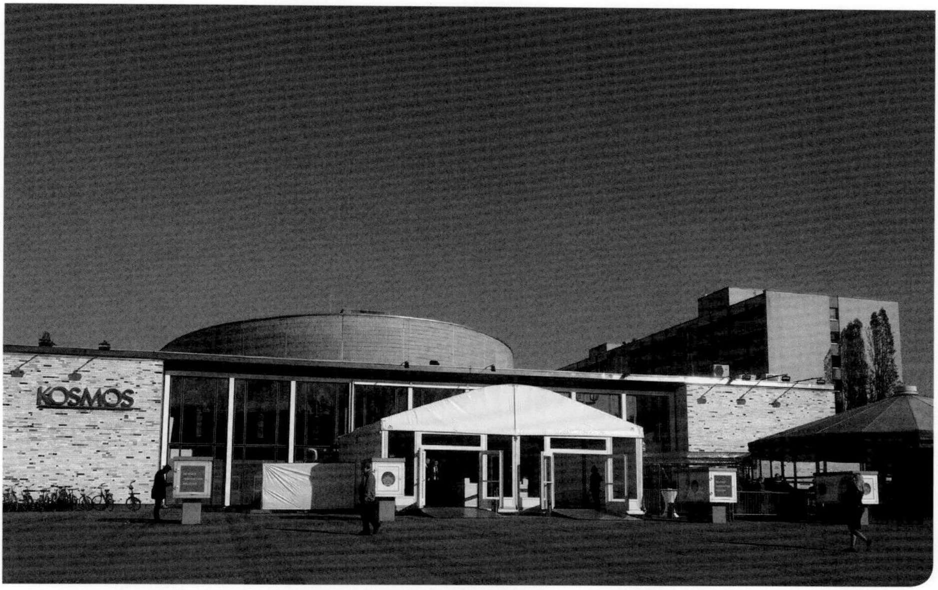

▲ *Venue of the World Health Summit 2017: Kosmos Berlin*

The Venue

The ninth World Health Summit took place at the Kosmos, Berlin. The venue was the largest and most popular film theatre in the former GDR. Today it's a popular public location. I had never been there before.

After passing the entrance security the participants reached the circular lobby around the main hall, decorated with science posters, seats, buffets and cafés, a perfect area for networking. I was very much impressed by the brandnew World Health Summit IT Spot, four monitor screens with graphics processing live social media data on the summit. One of the screens showed the most twittered tweeds from participants of the summit. Around the circular lobby smaller movie theatre rooms located the workshops.

The Program

This summit offered 47 events of three different categories: Keynote speeches, panel discussions and workshops. Every event on the summit was scheduled for one and a half hour. Central topics in 2017 were Health Policy in the G7/G20, Global Health Security, Healthy and Resilient Cities, Big Data, Vaccine Research and Development and Strenghtening Innovation and Health Systems in Africa.

For me the most interesting event was the panel discussion on global health security with chair Wolfgang Ischinger, chairman of the Munich Security Conference. The speakers Peter Albiez (CEO, Pfizer Germany), Richard Hatchett (CEO, Coalition for Epidemic Prepardness Innovation), Lord Paul Boateng (Member of the House of Lords,

UK), Peter Salama (Executive Director WHO) and Laurie Garrett (Council of Foreign Relations, USA) discussed the role of the WHO and its commitment to strengthen its emergencies programs and the world`s initiatives to prepare for the next pandemic.

Questions like "Are we doing enough?" and "Have the European Union and Germany found their role in the global health security?" were discussed vividly. The panel agreed, that international collaboration is the key to find more effective ways to respond to pandemics like Ebola. Different opinions persisted on the role every state should play in a better working health system.

This event looked also at the real value of private giving, the benefits in comparison to other sources of funding: a big challenge for the work and budget of the WHO. One percent of the richest people in the world can influence the future of diseases. The Bill & Melinda Gates Foundation served as an example for that. For many illnesses that afflict the world's poorest people, future funding is uncertain.

Lessons Learned

The World Health Summit is a perfect forum for discussing and networking – not only for experienced professionals from every field in the healthcare spectrum. There were more students than I expected. Every participant had a rather bulky sign attached to his neck with his name and occupation, making it quite easy to address questions or start a conversation. It seemed somehow like a class reunion, since many of the participants apparently knew each other form previous summits.

The World Health Summit offers an excellent platform to learn, advocate and act. The organizers integrate students, men and women, by cooperating with the program Young Physician Leaders, a worldwide network of selected students with medical background.

The World Health summit's organization is excellent as comprehensive signposting, the at all times operational internet access, the fast security check at the entrance and the perfectly distributed rich buffets show. Great service: All events are available as video-streams.

At least one wish from a first year student for the next World Health Summit 2018: better information about international student organizations and creating a platform to student organizations for informing and presenting themselves.

(Hanna Sendler)

M8 Alliance Declaration World Health Summit 2017, Berlin

Health is a political choice

Global health is increasingly shaped in the political arena. For the first time the heads of state of the G20 included priority global health issues in their final declaration. Health is recognized as a central piece of the Sustainable Development Agenda 2030 and it is now a regular feature at the UN General Assembly. Many regional political bodies are engaging to improve health whilst city initiatives for health are gaining in relevance. The member states of the WHO have elected a new Director General with a strong commitment to the right of all people to Universal Health Coverage (UHC) and to gender equity. At the same time global solidarity for health is challenged by a wave of populism. This year's World Health Summit (WHS) sends a strong message that determined political leadership is required to counteract forces that endanger global health progress.

The rich discussions at the World Health Summit 2017 lead us to highlight the need for action in six key areas of global health:

1. Commitment to Strong and Reliable Governance

The world needs strong global health institutions to set norms and standards, respond to outbreaks and to protect and support the most vulnerable. Their work needs the support of decision makers at the highest level and it is essential that health remains a key issue in major political fora such as the G7 and the G20 and in all regional organizations. Topics such as health security, antimicrobial resistance and the health impact of climate change, "One Health", "Health in all Policies" reach far beyond the health sector and need the involvement of heads of government and other stakeholders. Interdisciplinary collaboration is the critical factor – all stakeholders from academia, the private sector, civil society and politics have to work together. Governments have to coordinate their activities, support international cooperation and strengthen the World Health Organization (WHO). The Sustainable Development Goals have provided the road map for action.

The M8 Alliance calls on the countries hosting the next G7 and G20 summits and holding the presidencies of key regional organizations to include global health challenges on their agendas and to make the political choices required to ensure the implementation of the 2030 SDG agenda.

2. Commitment to Ensure Global Health Security

The world is not yet ready to respond sufficiently to a major pandemic threat, despite a range of new initiatives which have been created to support greater health security for all. The joint global effort to implement the International Health Regulations (IHR) must continue with vigor and strong financial support – from both donor and domestic resources. Investments in science and innovation as well as in public health institutions and capacity are critical. This requires synergies between national, regional and global action, between public and private actors and between development und humanitarian organizations.

The M8 Alliance calls on decision makers to maintain and strengthen their investment in health security, especially the implementation of the IHR. This must include ensuring the safety of health and humanitarian workers in war and conflict zones. Investing in resilient health systems and capacity at community level is one of the best approaches to ensure greater safety and reduce vulnerability.

3. Commitment to Healthy and Resilient Cities

Cities are becoming transformative drivers of sustainable development and key actors in global health. Their challenge is to act for health locally and integrate health into urban planning, housing investment and social policy decisions as cities continue to grow and change. Urban populations face many health risks, among them pollution, noise, overcrowding, traffic, insufficient access to drinking water and sanitary facilities, crime, and infectious disease. The NCD pandemic will only be resolved if there is also determined action at the city level. The M8 Alliances welcomes the increasing number of city initiatives and networks that support health and calls on Mayors to give particular attention to the social determinants of health and their impact on the next generation of children and young people.

4. Commitment to Responsible Approaches to Big Data

Data are increasingly a cornerstone of the healthcare in all sectors including industry and its value is rising exponentially. It documents everything from blood pressure readings, wearables, sensors and treatment outcomes, surgical records to insurance claims, immunization histories, patient demographics and receipts of payment. Big Data and artificial intelligence can bridge the gap between healthcare delivery and population health and improve many health outcomes through enhanced methods of research. The digital future of health has only just begun and in many cases outpaces the policy responses.

The M8 Alliance calls on international organizations and on policy makers to prioritize the digital potential of health systems and to

rapidly and systematically address the ethical, commercial, regulatory and technical challenges that come with this change.

5. Commitment to Research, Innovation and Development

Progress in global health is driven by great scientific progress and innovation in health research. Investing in basic research, science and technology is a game changer in all areas – In global health the development of vaccines offers the best means for controlling, eliminating and eradicating dangerous communicable pathogens. Intensified global efforts to step up vaccine research and development are therefore essential and a range of new initiatives – such as GAVI and CEPI – support the move in this direction. Important initiatives are also emerging to address the challenge of antimicrobial resistance. Part of such an effort must be the support to institution and capacity building in the global South and strong cooperation networks that span the globe. The support of digitalization is a key component of any such strategy.

The M8 Alliance calls on countries, private sector actors and international organizations to significantly step up their investment in innovation, science and technology, including implementation sciences, interdisciplinary and translational work as well as technology transfer.

6. Commitment to Innovation and Health Systems Strengthening in Africa

Achieving the Sustainable Development Goals will require significant innovations regarding how investments and partnerships are developed with low and middle income counties around the world, especially in Africa. This includes information sharing and knowledge exchange. A new generation of well-trained scientists and health professionals stands ready to contribute if there are institutions within which they can work and serve. Domestic investment will play an ever more important role – yet cooperation among African countries as in other regions of the world will be more important than ever before in order to muster the still scarce resources.

The M8 Alliance calls on professional organizations to actively contribute to new models of institution building and professional development to promote indigenous capacity in science and technology. Strategies to develop a highly competent health workforce, managing work force migration and circulation, involvement of Diasporas of professionals and scientists will gain in relevance. First successes in Africa show that progress is possible – they must be stepped up and supported.

The M8 Alliance renews its full commitment to support goal 3 of the

Sustainable Development Goals which aims to: "Ensure healthy lives and promote wellbeing for all at all ages." We call on heads of state and government to invest in people and to ensure that no one is left behind.

The M8 Alliance commits to the transformative approach of the Sustainable Development Goals. Success in SDG goal 3 will be achieved in a cross sectoral approach involving many of the other SDGs. We call on politicians to make the political choice for health.

World Health Summit:

The World Health Summit is one of the world's most prominent strategic forums for global health. The interdisciplinary event takes place within an atmosphere of academic freedom and is the premiere international platform for exploring strategic developments and decisions in the area of healthcare.

Every October, internationally renowned leaders and representatives from the sciences, politics, business, and civil society travel to Berlin for the World Health Summit to discuss the latest challenges facing medical research and healthcare. The World Health Summit enjoys the high patronage of German Chancellor Angela Merkel, the President of the French Republic Emmanuel Macron and European Commission President Jean-Claude Juncker

M8 Alliance:

The M8 Alliance of Academic Health Centers, Universities and National Academies is a unique collaborative network and think tank, made up of leading international medical universities, research institutions and all National Academies of medicine and science, the InterAcademy Partnership (IAP). The M8 Alliance was founded in 2009 at the inaugural World Health Summit, and has provided an outstanding academic foundation ever since.

The M8 Alliance currently has 25 members based in 18 different countries, all of which are committed to improving global health and working with political and economic decision-makers to develop science-based solutions to health challenges worldwide. The M8 Alliance promotes the translation of research from bench to bedside to population health, as well as the transformation of current medical care approaches to treating the ill by creating healthcare systems aimed at the effective prevention of disease at the global level.

5. Global Health Security

Timo Ulrichs

In preparation of the World Health Summit, a working group convened at the Command Staff College (Führungsakademie der Bundeswehr) in Hamburg to discuss the emerging scientific field of Global health and security. The working group consisted of representatives from the Harvard Medical School, Boston; the King's College, London; the Center for Global Health Engagement at the Uniformed Services University; the Hertie School of Governance, Berlin; and the Akkon University for Human Sciences, also Berlin.

To reveal the relationship between health, security and peace, definitions of each subject were elaborated including negative descriptions (health = absence of disease or infirmity (see also WHO definition); security = absence of threat; peace = absence of violence). To further define the new field of global health security, it was helpful to look into the basic documents like the WHO Constitution of 1946:

"The health of all peoples is fundamental to the attainment of peace and security and is dependent on the fullest cooperation of individuals and states."

The working group consisted of representatives from politics, education and training, health and medicine, academia and military. Thus, it was necessary to not only develop a working definition of global health security (GHS), but also to localize the new joint scientific and research field among the respective own background.

From the military and political (security sector) perspective, GHS means that the security sector provides the framework for global health workers to fulfill their tasks for health globally (fig. 1).

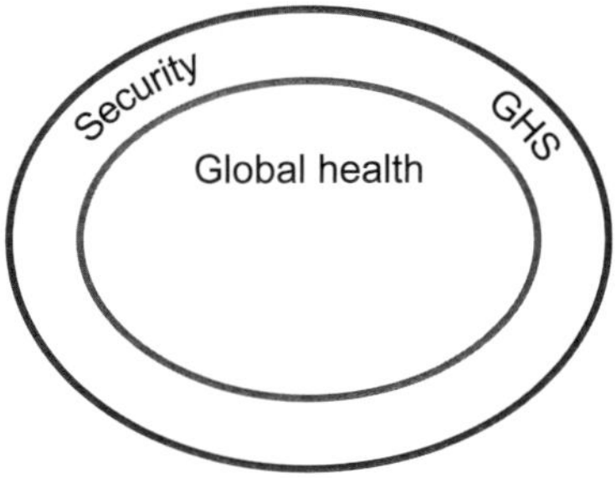

From the medical and health perspective (health sector), GHS is one of various projects/fields within global health and deals with securing health (care systems) against outer threats like epidemics, military conflicts, even non-communicable diseases (fig. 2).

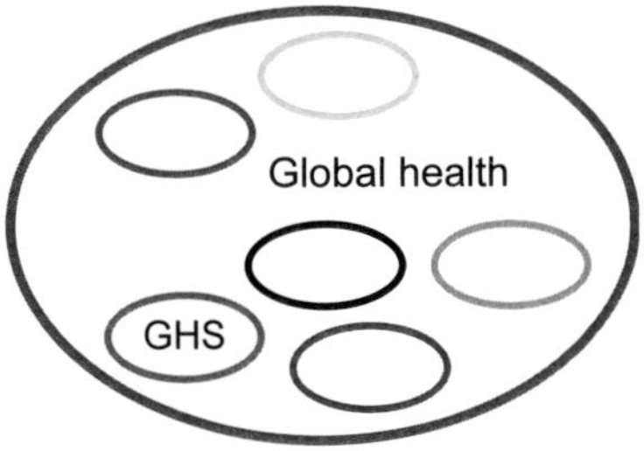

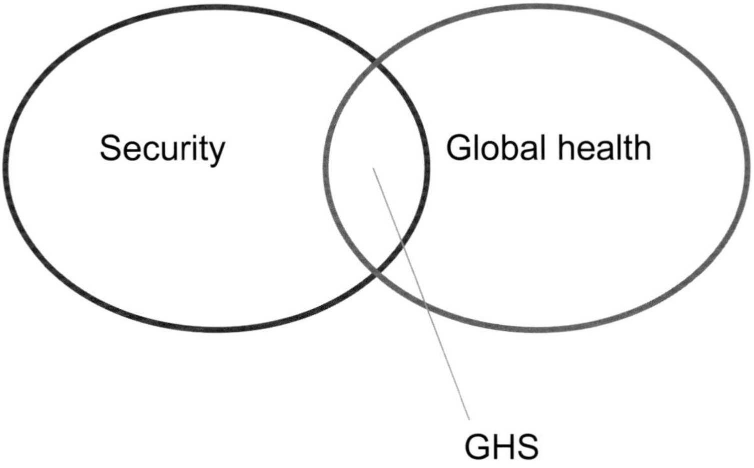

However, to bring together people interested in global (in the sense of comprehensive, worldwide) questions regarding security and health from the above-mentioned fields, it is necessary to define questions of mutual interest and to develop a work plan to answer them (fig. 3).

In addition, in order to avoid a too narrow description of activities, it might be necessary establish GHS as own research field interacting with both the security and the health sector independently. Thus, a multisectoral and multidisciplinary approach is needed.

The working group organized the session on Global health security at the World Health Summit and re-convened in the week after to finally discuss definition of GHS, tasks, challenges and opportunities of the topic. Its efforts resulted in the adoption of a white paper about GHS which is attached to this chapter.

After agreeing on the contents of the white paper, the working group renamed itself into Global Health Security Alliance and established a website, www.glohsa.com. The following activities were establishing a collaboration with the Munich Security Conference, submitting GHS topics into various conferences and congresses and working on teaching and training tools on GHS.

Concept paper on the future of global health security

Introduction

Events like the 2014 Ebola outbreak and Cholera epidemics in Yemen and Haiti, have highlighted how crises that outstrip health system capacities can fuel instability as well as prompt security sector interventions. Likewise, insecurity from armed conflict, disasters, and mass migration can destroy health systems and reverse global health achievements.

The recognition of this interplay between security and health has given rise to the concept of "global health security" (GHS). To date, efforts in this arena have largely focused on promoting states' capabilities to detect and respond to infectious disease outbreaks.

Progress in this regard notwithstanding, threats to global health security have escalated over the past five years. Namely, the destruction of health systems from armed conflict including in Syria, Iraq and Yemen, climate change-derived health impacts, and the rise of antimicrobial resistant pathogens all threaten future health security crises with global repercussions.

Over the last year, discussions regarding GHS threats have gained prominence in forums from the Munich Security Conference to the 2017 G7 and G20 meetings. The urgency of these threats, as well as the recognition that addressing them may require joint efforts among security, development and health actors, provide an opportunity to consider key issues and challenges with respect to the future direction of this enterprise.

Aims

In October 2017, the Bundeswehr Command and Staff College facilitated a workshop on the future of global health security, convening experts in security policy, global health, military medicine and foreign affairs. Workshop participants considered three core questions:

1. What should the next generation of global health security efforts emphasize?
2. What should the role of non-health sectors, particularly the security sector be in promoting global health security?
3. How should goals be defined and a Global Health Security enterprise, with its plurality of stakeholders and actors be governed?

This Concept paper outlines these deliberations, and reflects feedback received during private consultations with experts as well as in public forums including the Berlin World Health Summit 2017 and a Hertie School of Governance panel discussion.

A more detailed white paper elaborating on the ideas presented here is forthcoming.

Definition

Initial workshop discussions focused on generating a definition of global health security that distinguishes it from related concepts like global health and health system strengthening by explicitly connecting it with notions of security. The definition generated by workshop participants is as follows:

"Global Health Security is the collective ability to mitigate health threats that have the potential to destabilize societies, states and regions. The goal of Global Health Security is to establish resilient health systems in order to promote peace and security for all."

Features of this definition that appealed to participants included:

- its emphasis on the interconnectedness between security and health requiring a multi-sectoral approach
- its focus on health system resilience as integral to the concept of global health security
- its explicitness about the collective responsibility of global health security being a public good as such not rivalrous and not exclusive requiring the exercise of public authority at national and international level
- the notion that global health security promotion is a proactive enterprise about threat mitigation, rather than one that concerns crisis response alone

What should the next generation of GHS efforts emphasize?

Fragile States, specifically conflict affected states and war zones with damaged or collapsed health systems are the most likely places for epidemics and other GHS threats to emerge. To date there has been little focus on developing strategies for protecting and recovering health systems in fragile settings, in some cases because of concerns about the political dynamics of doing so. In fact, there are currently no widely accepted methods or indicators to identify vulnerabilities to health systems or monitor health systems at risk of disruption.

Furthermore, most states in acute or chronic crisis lack some or all of the critical health subsystems necessary to robustly address emerging threats to populations health. For example, animal disease surveillance and response subsystems to detect emerging zoonotic threats remain poorly resourced and integrated into disease surveillance systems in most nations. Participants recommended:

1. Developing and monitoring indicators of threats and disruptions to national health systems. These indicators should:

a) Enable domestic and international stakeholders to anticipate and identify significant early trends that suggest health system's risk of dysfunction.

b) Identify existing and emerging vulnerabilities for investment to mitigate risk and increase resilience (e.g. animal health surveillance, diagnostic and response systems must be strengthened to address zoonosis).

c) Suggest targets for intervention of international stakeholders to act in response to acutely dysfunctional and/or critically-underperforming systems.

2. Developing ethical and legal frameworks to inform decision making related to supporting health systems in fragile situations. This framework must reflect International Humanitarian Law and human rights law and address salient concerns of involved state and non-state actors in relation to providing access to health care, health system protection, addressing corruption, and potential disruption or displacement of state (nation) health resources by external actors.

What should the role of non-health sectors, particularly the security sector be in promoting global health security?

The ambition of Global Health Security is to bring together critical interdisciplinary actors to protect threatened health systems, mitigate the impacts of health system collapse, reduce the chances of global health security repercussions, and develop health system resilience to prevent future threats. National and international security organizations have historically responded to crises and disasters. The UN Interagency Standing Committee's guidelines on their roles and responsibilities have guided their engagement in these efforts. With the rise of the security paradigm in health, the engagement of the security sector in global health is becoming more frequent. Participants acknowledged a range of concerns about the increased involvement of security actors in global health. Normative standard development for the ethical application of security organization capabilities would be enhanced, participants felt, by delineating the most appropriate security sector capabilities relevant to GHS and defining threshold criteria for their use. In addition, participant recommendations included:

1. Articulate areas for investment of security resources in building capacity and advancing resilient national and regional health

systems to mitigate risk of potential or emerging health threats.

2. Practice GHS responses through multi-sectoral international exercises. One goal of these exercises should be to build a more integrated response between national and international security organizations and health system stakeholders.

3. Studying the health, social, economic, security and political outcomes and impacts of security sector engagement in Global Health Security.

How should the Global Health Security enterprise, with its plurality of stakeholders and actors be governed?

Global health security is a collective responsibility to secure health systems that support not only human life but also the foundation for a "healthy functioning state". As such governance from the local to the international level is required to coordinate and facilitate GHS efforts. Among the international organizations, the World Health Organization (WHO) with the power vested in it by its Constitution and the International Health Regulations, is uniquely well positioned to coordinate and promote GHS efforts. Recognizing the need for the WHO and others to effectively collaborate, participants recommend the following actions:

1. Enhancing coordination among UN agencies and other health authorities to support WHO securing threatened health systems prior to crisis as outlined in the Sendai Framework.

2. Establish a formal United Nations Security Council (UNSC) subsidiary body to first advise the UNSC on Global Health issues and second to coordinate responses with WHO and other relevant GHS entities, if necessary.

3. Global Health Security is best served by effective governance from sovereign states working through whole-of-government mechanisms. Responsive international private and public support for integrated stateled efforts before, during, and after health crises is critical to effectively and efficiently build sustained functioning health systems. When states are unable to lead health crisis responses, every effort should be made to support reestablishment of legitimate governing authority.

Deliberations of the Global Health Security Alliance Workshop

Bundeswehr Command & Staff College
Hamburg, Germany
October, 2017

Global Health Security Alliance (GloHSA)
www.glohsa.com
info@glohsa.com